D1568764

A Proper Knowledge

A Proper Knowledge

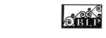

MICHELLE LATIOLAIS

BELLEVUE LITERARY PRESS
NEW YORK

First published in the United States in 2008 by
Bellevue Literary Press
New York

FOR INFORMATION ADDRESS:
Bellevue Literary Press
NYU School of Medicine
550 First Avenue
OBV 640
New York, NY 10016

This book was published with the generous support of
Bellevue Literary Press's founding donor the Arnold Simon Family Trust
and the Bernard & Irene Schwartz Foundation.

Library of Congress Cataloging-in-Publication Data

Latiolais, Michelle.
A proper knowledge / Michelle Latiolais. —1st ed.
p. cm.
1. Psychiatrists—Fiction 2. Sisters—Death—Fiction.
3. Autism—Research—Fiction. 4. Self-actualization (Psychology)—Fiction.
5. Psychological fiction. I. Title.
PS3562.A7585P76 2008   813'.54—dc22   2008006363

Book design and type formatting by Bernard Schleifer
Manufactured in the United States of America
ISBN 978-1-934137-11-6
FIRST EDITION
1 3 5 7 9 8 6 4 2

For
Michael Barsa
and
Keith Weitzman

for their compassion to others

. . . and [with] all similar children there needs to be genuine care and kindness if one wants to achieve anything at all. These children often show a surprising sensitivity to the personality of the teacher. However difficult they are even under optimal conditions, they can be guided and taught, but only by those who give them true understanding and genuine affection, people who show kindness towards them and, yes, humour. The teacher's underlying emotional attitude influences, involuntarily and unconsciously, the mood and behaviour of the child. Of course, the management and guidance of such children essentially requires a proper knowledge of their peculiarities as well as genuine pedagogic talent and experience. Mere teaching efficiency is not enough (48).

—*Autism and Asperger Syndrome*, edited by Uta Frith

Stan engines into Luke's office, his legs pistoning, fanatical, fueled by something seemingly unstoppable and mechanical, and so frightening—and frightening anew each time, Luke must admit—because each time Luke is alarmed and he knows it registers in his eyes and body until the physician arrives on board and he remembers who he is in this equation called doctor and patient.

"Stan, hey, how're you, guy?" but Luke doesn't wait for an answer, doesn't not wait, either, but, rather understands the continuum within which at any point in time an exchange with Stan is registering and being responded to, language and time not so much in constant shuffle as in constant deliberate reconfigurative negotiation.

"You feel the earthquake yesterday, buddy?" Luke asks, getting up from his chair and coming around his desk. He hunkers down near Stan to see if he won't make eye contact. Luke is six four, and even halved he is still taller than most of his charges.

Stan pulls the juice tin of colored pencils down one side of the low child's table, then across its lower ledge, then pushes the tin up to the top left-hand corner. He selects a pencil from the forty-five that are there, the same green pencil—*vert vif*—every session, then moves the tin counterclockwise back to its original position.

"In the morning, yesterday, the earth moved, jolted. You draw that for me, Stan? You give me a sense of what that felt like for you?" Luke pauses. He looks at Stan's thin, finely boned face, the huge eyes full of intelligence, perception, ferocity. Luke likes Stan's stylish eyeglasses, wonders absently what they cost, the blue frames with the snazzy ultra-thin line of red running across the top. "But I'd rather you just talked to me, buddy," he says, knowing the minute Stan does speak, Luke will have to work hard and fast at the sorting out, the putting together—is that a sentence from *The Lion King* or from *The Manchurian Candidate*? Luke stands up and shakes out his legs. His knees ache. He is better and better at racketball and this makes him unhappy, this being more skillful at something in the company of men alone—how regressive is that!—and the four tall, claustrophobic walls, his disorientation more and more often—Where is the door? How do I get out of here?—the balls strafing past his ears maniacally, so how he's gotten better might be a mystery, but it isn't. He's madder, more aggressive; that passage to "better," he'd rather have no part of. He supposes there are women who play racketball, but his reach at six four is expansive and he'd be wary of clipping her with a racket. Anyway, that's not exactly what he wants, a racketball partner.

He leans back against one of the chairs in front of his desk. He loves Stan's straight blond hair, which is left to fall to his shoulders. He already looks like a graduate student, Luke thinks, but an ethereal one. Stan positions the pencil carefully in his fingers, pulling his own thumb farther down the pencil's shaft. He then smoothes the air above the paper for several seconds with the backs of his hands. He steps away, steps forward, and begins. He draws swiftly, adroitly, his hand flying two inches above the page; he pulls a line down left, then extends it farther, tweaks a detail in the upper right corner, worries something dead center, eddying the pencil around and around—it might be a Giacometti face—but there is absolutely no mark on the paper anywhere.

Something occurs to Luke that has not before: Stan is tall for seven, beautifully proportioned, as elegant as a giraffe, but he will only lean over so far. The child's table is low for him, and Luke has never seen Stan of his own accord, or willingly, take to a chair.

"Hey, buddy, let's set you up here." Luke drags a chair away from the front of his desk and clears away the picture of Sadie, the smaller picture of Man and his man, a rock formation off the coast of Cornwall, England, and a silver letter opener which should not have been out during a session anyway. He leans across his desk and slides them into a drawer. He pushes his blotter aside and then pulls from the child's table the pad Stan has been gesturing over. Luke positions it carefully on the desk. "Bring your pencil, guy. Draw here, okay? The desk will be a better height for you to work on."

Stan doesn't turn around to face Luke or to acknowledge what Luke has suggested and now arranged for him. "You know you don't have to sit in a chair," Luke urges. Stan stands very still, a small, narrow statue; there is a tremendous, calamitously still anger rigidifying his body, and then the anger is kinetic and he begins to turn, his arms held close to his body, turning, turn-ing, dervishing, his arms opening to maintain his balance, and Luke knows he must wait, maybe five, maybe ten, maybe fifteen minutes before Stan stops, and that, in fact, it is therapeutic for Stan to twirl, that he'll be calmer afterward, his coordination better.

Luke walks around his desk and sits in his chair, which he swivels to face Stan and then swivels around to gaze out the window. He's done a stupid thing by changing the location of the drawing pad within the same session. He should have made his observation and then next session have set the pad on a higher surface, perhaps even have gotten a drafting table. There is a lot of room in Luke's office, a broad expanse of carpet, which he has deliberately left open. Furniture is a kind of restraint, particularly unwelcome to boys, and the fewer obstacles for children to hit up against, to garner bruises, the better, but he wants a taller table for Stan. There's plenty of room. Stan may never use it, but Luke would like to see anyway. Luke used to pride himself a bit on his ability to read his patients' bodies, the occult way these bodies communicate need, but he doesn't much anymore. Luck is luck, he knows now, and you can't take much credit for it. He'd had luck with patients; that is all it had been, other than it had led him to think of himself as having some proper knowledge of his patients—or the ability to gather it. A fool's paradise. God, what a fool's paradise, he thinks, watching the twirling blur of Stan before him. He realizes he is also dis-tracted today by the prospect of the christening he must attend. He finds it somewhat unbelievable that the middle of the day on a Friday was chosen for this event. Glen and Naila are both doctors, and so are many of their friends, including Luke. What were they thinking? But then Luke thinks *inconvenient* Glen's middle name, and Naila far too gentle for her own good. Luke, he says to himself, focus, for God's sake, though now, because of Stan's twirling, he will have several minutes before his attention is really needed.

He moves his chair slowly around and pulls Sadie's face from his desk drawer and puts it before him on his desk, just beyond the blotter, where it always is. Of the doctors who had treated his sister, he would have killed them before hearing of any such inattentiveness. He could kill them now for what they'd done, or not done for Sadie, the lackadaisical asses—and he no better.

"Spit your shit, Mucus Lucas," he hears her say. He runs his finger down her nose, a long straight nose, rather flat, like their father's. Sadie looks—or looked—like him, much more than Luke does, the long oval face, angular jaw, the deep-set flashing eyes, and perfect, perfect teeth behind full lips, though Sadie's lips rarely stopped quivering, working something over and over, always working something. Luke doesn't brood on his and Sadie's father much—he doesn't have much to brood on, a few photographic portraits and one candid snap his mother kept—keeps—among the orchard of framed pictures on the baby grand, a Moroccan leather jewelry box, his military brush-es, the diploma for his Ph.D. in anthropology. Luke thinks there are different types of absences, that his father's is an absence that merely deepened, intensified, became the paragon of what it always was to begin with. In his mind, Sadie is a hotter, more constant absence, a presence really, a standard by which he works each day, a measure of his existence as a doctor. She's been dead twenty-one years, diagnosed schizophrenic at the age of eleven, and he hears every day in his mind's ear what the doctors heard, the odd phrases, the difficult and uncomfortable questions, the vocabulary: "Clues, why do you need clues? Are you in a maze? Don't ask Maisie; she's being trussed for supper. I certainly did not teach her to be food. That's what the word *clue* means, a ball of yarn. How do you thread it through a conch shell? Bulls are vegetarian; the Greeks made the Minotaur eat human flesh because that's all they fed him."

Years after the diagnosis, but within a few days of becoming a doctor, Luke petitioned to see Sadie's files. He remembers sitting at his mother's house, on the patio, the beautiful terraced garden before him, and the huge manila envelope across his lap. He sat awhile, listening to the birds and to the low whir of traffic a few blocks away on San Vicente Boulevard. A garden spider hung in its intricate web not two feet from him. He wasn't afraid. That wasn't it. He knew pretty much what was there, what he'd find. It was the exhaustion of grief; it was finding enough energy to turn the envelope over, to finger his way inside; it was the exhaustion of knowing too unalterably what he would find. "High-functioning autistic children are often fact obsessed, their interests tending toward the technological and scientific. Sadie [and then oddly her last name had been inked out] shows little if any interest in the aforementioned disciplines, and though her grasp of Syrian and Greek mythologies is noteworthy, I suggest her interest in these products of prerational culture borders on reification and is thus an extension of her delusional world. Advise a course of psychotropics."

The doctor's signature was unreadable, but Luke could reach out with a pen and reproduce its hieroglyphics in the light of his office without looking, without thinking; like Stan, Luke muses, he could carve that signature into the air before his face, the snarl of letters there, always, and just as much not there, the phantom of a consulting doctor who helped seal his sister's fate.

Luke hears even now, each day, what the attending doctors heard, hears what provoked them to call in the expert, hears what they sensed was autism, the immense loneliness of Sadie's verbal barrage, its learnedness, the obsessive intensity of her fascination with mythology. At least those early doctors struggled to maintain a sense of Sadie as able, extraordinary, "highfunctioning" a bromidic epithet they strove for. Instead, one unreadable signature—this last doctor called in—and Sadie was drugged into compliance for a disease she didn't have, entombed so elegantly, she disappeared beyond the reach of language or nurture. Hakuna Matata, Luke thinks derisively, no worries for the rest of your days—ten milligrams of Prolixin Decanoate—though to be fair to Disney, the film doesn't exactly end up propounding that sensibility, no worries. But why are the zebras always dancing in *The Lion King*? You'd think the high visibility of lions feasting on zebra haunches would contraindicate *dancing*—

Luke swivels completely around and sees that Stan's eyes are beginning to emerge, to focus, to peer out from the revolutions of his head. Sooner than ever before, Stan slows and finally twirls one last time and stops. Stan returns to the child's table and rolls the page up the tablet of paper. He pivots swiftly and then stares straight ahead, past Luke's head, as though just beyond the window is inspiration, some meteorological accumulation that compels him to draw.

"Because it's your responsibility," Stan says blandly. "It means you're a baboon and I'm not."

Luke knows the lines from *The Lion King*, Stan speaking the part of the baboon who augurs, who learns from his bones and coconuts that Simba, the heir apparent, is alive, ashamed of returning to the Pride Lands to take up his role as king. Stan, Luke surmises, is lecturing him, shaming him into some course of action—or *out* of that course, more than likely.

"Creepy little monkey," Luke says, though he usually hesitates to respond in lines from the two movies Stan perseverates. Luke makes his voice sound like Stan's bland monotone.

"The question is, Who are you?" Stan shouts furiously, his

hand sketching in the air above the paper, the *vert vif* pencil moving rapidly, expertly, then pausing startlingly, gently stroking in some affect or expression—a dark iris?, or perhaps a cheek in shadow?—and then, just as abruptly, his hand returns to its previous fervor which now intensifies to a mad slashing . . . and all of it in the air, unreadable on paper.

The jacaranda is in bloom and the campus is purple-hued, beautiful. Luke is early. He walks toward Doheny Library with its Italianate architecture, at least he thinks it Italianate, the intricate brick and fretwork. He has never been to the chapel on the USC campus and he meanders a bit, the way one meanders on a campus, heading more vaguely than usual in a given direction. "Over there, behind Doheny, near Pioneer Hall," the student says, not looking at him, her straight blond hair tossed from her face. Annoyance? Attitude? Shyness? He can't tell. "I appreciate the help," he says. "God knows I do," and then she laughs a little, looking up at him.

"Later," she says. But there will be no later, Luke thinks a little meanly, looking across the rose garden blooming with red and yellow roses, or rather cardinal and gold, USC's colors. Chinatown is all Luke can ever see when he sees red and yellow together, and it doesn't matter which Chinatown—Los Angeles, San Francisco, New York—as every Chinatown has a Canton market with huge red-and-yellow plastic bags. *Later* might be Peking duck wrapped in crepes spread with plum sauce and long strips of scallion, the blond student across the table— annoyed, affected, shy, whatever it is she is! . . . But no, later he'll eat with his friends, the gang, his colleagues, his old classmate, this new baby. It will be fine, he thinks, good, other doctors, his friends, their company, their little one, fine, just fine, talking himself into it, though not sure why he is having to. His mother will be there, and Janey, and if lunch were just the three of them, he'd welcome the meal. But no, instead—strategically—he'll be seated near some poor sister or friend of a friend prevailed upon to entertain him. Maybe not today, Luke thinks to himself. Maybe today he'll just slip that little white card next to his mother and Janey, or next to Naila, though she'll now have the baby. Naila, what had she gotten herself into?

He traverses a wide old lane lined with magnolia trees, their dark green foliage dotted here and there with huge white flowers just beginning to open. He likes being back on a college campus, is reminded of how peaceful it can be, how inward-turning, and he is suddenly happy to be here to welcome this baby into the world—at least he's charging himself with the chore of being happy. He's actually never been to a christening, and he wonders if that is odd, unusual, a man thirty-seven years old attending his first. He supposes these ceremonies are most often familial and small, religiously intimate, or actually—he thinks—don't they usually take place during church services? Then he is angry again at the timing, not pleased that an appointment with Zeke had to be canceled, moved, and Zeke so closed down anyway, as if saying, Do anything you want to me; it doesn't matter. Which, of course, drove Luke to be particularly careful of him, to recognize and honor any expression of will he presented. And Zeke's will, as velleitous as it was, seemed at least inclined to therapy with Luke, something his sweet, careful parents had divined because Zeke—almost completely mute—would start to slowly rearrange their living room to look like Luke's office. Zeke had been a late child in a long, happy, though childless, marriage, and all he would have ever had to have done was whisper his desires for them to be instantly realized.

Luke looks up to see a very small structure nestled within a densely landscaped passage just beyond the lane. He isn't sure it can be anything but the chapel, but he isn't completely sure it's that, either, and no one stands outside loading a camera, a shoulder cranked up, talking on a cellular. He reaches the heavy wooden door and pulls it open slowly. It doesn't matter whether he is in the right place or not, because, regardless, he is drawn through the door, drawn through the curling ivy and flowers shrouding the entry and emanating into the sanctuary along the stone floors until the garlanded vines reach the few pews, up which they climb and circle. The chapel is as small as a bedroom, enshrouded, bowered. It seems at once enchanting and not at all enchanting. Luke is the only one here. Jesus Christ, he thinks, sitting down, and then he sees the tracery of vines across the back of the pew like a net beaded with blue flowers. How on earth is it all staying alive, unwilted? He looks down and sees flowers at the base of the pew in front of him, and on the inside of the leg, as though within some wooded nook where flowers might actually grow, protected from wind and the muzzles of deer. He leans out to see the aisle, and there, quietly, all along the floor stones to the font, someone has placed tufts of moss and gathers of vines. He starts looking very concertedly at this over-grown burrow, and more flowers emerge to his eye, small tied bundles on ledges beneath stained-glass windows and here and there along the pews, sweet william, rosemary, lavender. Were people to pick these up and hold them, take them? The most profuse display of flowers starts on the floor behind a table and entwines its way up the legs to spread, as though growing, around the guest registry. He tries to name these flowers but can't. Roses, those he knows, and hydrangeas, but there is a deep blue cattail of a flower, so many of these, and then a dense yellow broccoli he's never seen before.

"You should sign that, Luke," a woman's voice says softly, and he turns sharply to see his friend's wife, Naila, with her dark Egyptian eyes, smiling, holding her baby.

"Who did this?" he asks, standing up, walking to her, leaning to kiss her on the cheek. "The chapel, the flowers, it's kind of great."

"You think so?" she asks seriously, shifting the baby, and it is then that Luke sees the baby embowered, too, tiny roses around her face and across her tiny shoes.

"I do," he says. "Very much I do." Then a few people are entering and Luke shakes hands with his old classmate and congratulates him. Glen has wanted this for a long, long time, to be a father, and now it has happened, and Luke can see that Glen is already changed. It registers immediately with Luke, this chauvinism of a certain stripe, and he doesn't like it. He feels nasty for perceiving it, but the chauvinism is there, sharp and righteous. Oh, Glen, he thinks, you're in for some insights.

"Thank you for that amazing airplane, Luke," his friend says, holding his tie up and buzzing it about like a plane. "Where on earth did you find such a clever gift for a girl?"

Luke laughs in spite of himself—in spite of Glen. "New Jersey."

"What do you mean, New Jersey? You shop in New Jersey?" Glen pronounces the words with a kind of nasty incredulity.

Naila looks tired to Luke, the skin of her face a little blotchy, discolored. She puts her free hand on her husband's elbow. "It's so beautifully made," she says, "and wooden. Already I'm sick of luridly colored plastic objects."

Naila, Luke thinks, Naila. What are you doing with this jerk?

"New Jersey?" Glen repeats, not letting it go.

"One of Louise's favorite shops—and it just happens to be, of all places, in the Garden State. I have no idea how she knows about it," Luke says as pleasantly as he can muster. "You can ask her yourself."

"Luke," Naila begins quietly, "do you really like it? The chapel—"

"I think it's amazing."

"Glen thinks it's weird."

"If my baby were a rabbit, I'd even think it weird," Glen mumbles, turning around to greet other friends, more doctors, Luke thinks, than any one structure should be made to hold. Then Glen turns back to Luke abruptly. "See this one," Glen says, pointing at his baby in his wife's arms. "She's never going to need you, Luke. Never."

It's a showstopper, this comment, and for a minute there is a tableau vivant as everyone seems to stop, to become attendants at a baby christening. Even if this child did need him, Luke thinks, even if she did, he would not do that to Naila; he'd find a better doctor, one Glen wouldn't be right about. Luke sees that what's stunning about Glen's comment—and on this occasion and in this setting—is that it ignites the undergrowth, ignites what is beneath the joy and hope of almost any ceremony; for one hyper-still moment, fear takes a searing hold in all of them.

"How are you, Naila?" Luke asks to diffuse Glen's comment. "I know you had to be in bed for most of this."

"One issue after the other—but this makes me happy, our closest friends here, and I think the chapel looks lovely. I'm glad you think so, too. How's your mother?" Naila asks, but then she murmurs, smiling, "I guess all I need to do is wait to see."

"As only Louise can be seen," Luke says. "Who did it?" he asks again. "The chapel, the flowers, or greenery? . . . It's hard to know the right word."

"It cost a fortune," Naila says, and Luke laughs at this. For some reason, it makes him happy, Glen divested! and yet Glen had probably made Naila pay for it.

"Her name's Alice Samara and she does these . . ." and Naila's voice trails off. She twists her torso slowly from side to side, the baby quiet, mesmerized within the bower of her tiny roses.

"Installations?" Luke offers.

"Sort of, yes, I suppose, but this isn't that self-conscious, is it? Is it?" she asks him seriously, but doesn't wait for an answer. "They've done this book about her, or no, not about her, about the flowers—I guess she's fairly reclusive."

"She did this, too?" he asks, pointing to the bonnet and shoes.

"Everything."

Naila is drawn away and Luke moves to the guest registry, takes up the pen laid in its well, and leans down and enters his name on a pristine page. He draws a picture of a baby rabbit in a bonnet flying in a toy plane, its lop ears suspended in the wind. He takes some time refining the front paws and the very leafy carrots clutched within. He realizes someone stands behind him, waiting, a woman. He quickly pens in a pursuing Glen in a doctor's lab coat grasping a spray can. Luke tilts the book and writes "EXFOLIANT" boldly on the can. The drawing takes up the entire page and so he turns to a fresh one and presses the binding to keep the stiff page in place. He moves aside and hands the pen to her.

"I think I'll just have to sign my name." She feigns displeasure, and then, realizing that there is no place for her to put her purse, reaches up and hangs its thin gold chain over Luke's shoulder.

"Glen's sister," he says, as though making a wild guess, but he knows her name, had been at her wedding, had even gotten invited by her to the bachelorette party for Naila. She was flamboyant and statuesque, a mouth on her a mile wide. "What better way to hook you up," she'd said, and saying it she'd been mocking those who had tried to put women in Luke's way, and he'd liked her because of this, and because she could get Glen's goat like no one else.

"I prefer 'the proud aunt,'" she pronounces now, signing her name—"SHEILA!"—flashily across the page with her left hand, the book held down with her right. "One page per customer, Luke! You've set the standard." Luke sees that she wears two simple gold wedding bands on her right hand.

"What's that about?" he asks, pointing down at her hand, sorry the question flies before he can check himself. He realizes there have now been two marriages.

"Double indemnity . . . but then again . . ." and her voice trails off.

Some vague memory of her divorces comes to Luke, a nasty comment by Glen about her choice of men. Luke can't imagine Glen having much discernment that way, either, but just who Sheila might be attracted to is a mystery to Luke. She certainly had never tossed any looks his way, not that he thought of himself as a better choice. Still, he'd been here, and she was funny and smart, and a little disastrous, which he thought he might like. "Tell me," he says to change the subject, because really, in this setting, he just doesn't want to be thinking about Glen's sister right now, "what do you think of the chapel? Your brother dislikes it."

"So Glen is Glen. What are you going to do, pull his toenails out? Believe me, I tried that as a kid." She turns the registry back to Luke's drawing and laughs loudly, even a little wildly. To Luke, everyone seems to turn and stare. He works the chain of her purse off his shoulder and holds it out to her. "Thanks," he says, "now I'm in trouble."

"You did that on your own." She smiles. "Where's my brother—no, actually, where's your mother? I haven't seen her in forever," and just then Luke sees Louise appear through the door, her eyes alight, and Janey behind her in a white lace dress and combat boots, her hair only vaguely pink. "This is marvelous," his mother is saying. "Look at this—it's charming."

"For a rabbit," Glen says loudly.

Aren't you dependable, Glen, Luke thinks. His mother wears one of the suits he likes best on her, pink, with carved onyx buttons she'd bought years ago when his father was around and Louise and Luke had shuffled their despondent selves down to Mexico City to meet up with him, where he was resting from a dig and consulting at the museum. "Onyx!" his father had said, holding up one of the buttons. "In medieval Europe, they used to think you could see someone's soul in an onyx mirror," and neither Luke nor his mother had said anything in the cool damp of the museum basement, where they had joined him after their lunch and desultory shopping. Somehow whatever his father said, his unchanged tone, denied his daughter, Sadie, had ever existed. Only the deep past interested him, and it had taken Louise several years to have a suit made, the buttons pronounced upon, small portals to a possibility Louise didn't believe in. Luke kisses her on the forehead now and thumps Janey on hers. "What," he says, "you don't have dress shoes?"

"She looks spectacular, you philistine," his mother says, smiling. "Thank God."

Luke watches Janey gazing about the chapel, transfixed. "Geez Louise, look at this," she keeps saying, waving his mother over. "Isn't it fantastic!"

Luke waits for them to ask who has created this enforested

chapel, waits because he knows the answer, the name Alice Samara as immediately solid in his consciousness as the sense, too, that something has happened to this person, something incomprehensible, menacing. He remembers reading that in Nagasaki and Hiroshima, people had run and hidden themselves in trees and beneath bushes, had burrowed into the ground and covered themselves with leaves, and that later, the Japanese, so fastidious in their gardening, had reported plants growing strangely and flowers blossoming out of season, and in odd places, counter to their usual habits. This morning, standing in the chapel at USC, Luke feels assured that he is seeing the creation of cloister. This chapel, the way she has made it grow in upon itself, creating a space discrete from the walls, the growth looking for something, looking to protect something, someone. Luke sees what he sees, and he finds it fanciful—but also at once beautiful and fierce.

"How are you?" his mother asks, pulling him to a pew, and he knows she means the question, wants details, the truth. There are thin cushions sporadically placed along the pews, and Luke slides one over for Louise. He likes its old green velvet as creased as a turtle leg. "Hmm?" she intones when they are both seated. "How are you?"

"Why a Friday?" he asks beneath his breath, crossing his long legs and leaning toward Louise. "It's not particularly easy to re-schedule patients who thrive on an uninterrupted sequence. What's wrong with good old Sunday?"

"Naila doesn't look very good, does she?" Louise says, settling her purse beside her. "It will take awhile."

"Sex with Glen could take a lifetime to recover from."

"You know this?" she teases, glancing sideways at Luke. "Anyway, leave poor Glen alone. I hear he's a pretty fine surgeon."

"He is that, indeed—at least he's that." Luke reaches out to touch the ivy worked up under the curl of the pew back. The leaves are tiny, variegated, *real*, he seems to need to assure himself; they appear like wolf faces, their ears and muzzle. "What do you bet Naila stops practicing psychiatry?" he says to his mother, looking to where Naila stands, fatigue on her body as observable as a net. Luke likes Naila, and there had been a chance, years ago, but he hadn't taken her up on it, Naila too much like water to him, too forgiving, delicate. She frightened him because he had known himself well enough to know he needed someone sturdier, a foil, someone he wouldn't roll right over, and, typical of Naila, she had faded back as gently as she had ventured tentatively forward. That this had seemed like proof to Luke of what he feared, she not able to fight in some way for him, was a bit of youthful ego, and he knew this now, though not lamentably—she had still not been right for him. Then bam, Glen strode his gonads across the hospital cafeteria and gathered her right up and put her in his pocket, Naila's broad Egyptian hips just the easy passage his babies would need. More Glens in the world, that's what he wanted! But Naila's body held off something her heart hadn't thought to, and fetus after fetus arrived unimpeded and months too early. Every bit of glad-handing Glen had ever done came to bear on Naila's body, every doctor within Glen's broad righteous reach who knew anything at all about natural habitual abortion— about inhospitable wombs. Luke had watched from afar, thinking cancer in Naila's future as sure as anything, her immune system shut down even more than most women's when pregnant, a cocktail of drugs as newly minted as this morning. Jesus, Naila, Luke thinks. Jesus.

His mother leans her head into him, her platinum hair in its perfectly done French twist, and says quietly, "Seems like psychiatry would be a better area to take a break from than surgery, yes?" Luke doesn't answer at first. He has an impossible time taking a vacation, let alone a break, and over the years— and perhaps fueled by guilt—he has stopped taking more than a day here or there. Just getting these hours in the middle of today has been difficult. His mother has never worked in any professional capacity and there is a range of experiences she has never had and can't very accurately imagine herself into. Luke knows Louise can imagine Naila at home with babies; she cannot imagine a situation where Naila is needed just as much, where Naila is just as central, a practice with patients waiting in over-stuffed chairs, glancing with every noise toward Naila's door. In his mother's generation—or maybe it's just Louise—men are the essential professionals, the ones counted on for work; women come and go, fill in at best. She wouldn't say women are less expert, just less reliable, and their professional lives secondary—they do precisely what Naila has done, have babies, and then take care of them, as they should. "It's just a break," Louise says to him, working to cheer him, enunciating a defense he would more usually be enunciating to her.

"She won't be taking a break, Mother," Luke says. "Mark my words."

Their attention is drawn to the front of the chapel, to the slender stone font twisted in ivy and white roses. Glen has taken the baby into his arms and is cooing loudly to her, squishing her up into his face. Louise says quietly, seriously—she is looking at Naila bereft of her child—"I always do mark your words, Luke. But it's what she's chosen—it's what she seems to want."

Maybe, he thinks, maybe. How would you sort out all the conditioning a person undergoes from some actual individual desire? Of course, it couldn't be done, and with Naila, she would more than likely articulate and then argue beautifully her "choices," and she would insist—though there would be no clamor in her voice—that they *were* choices. Luke realizes that he's looking yet again at the chapel, and at the vines and flowers netting them all together. It could be a kind of fort this Alice Samara has created, a small green secrecy within a garden that a child finds and hides in. "It's very striking," isn't it?" his mother asks, regarding him closely, and then she adds quietly, "Glen isn't the worst choice Naila could have made. You know that."

But Luke doesn't think he does know that. Glen is a contract Naila has chosen to make with her life, and she's not the first woman he's seen do this, and for children, and their nurture. He supposes there is an issue upon which Glen has made a contract, too, and that is that the children will always come before him, before his and Naila's relationship. This all seems destined for disaster, Luke thinks, or at least affairs and divorces. There's something right about it—if we were still struggling to survive the primordial swamp—and something deeply wrong, too, now that we're not. But he's not going to win hearts and minds bringing it up much.

Janey tumbles over Luke's shoes, a big joke, arms flailing, and then settles on the other side of Louise. "Hey, 'What's up, Doc?'" she says, Bugs Bunny–style. She sits on the edge of the seat, her legs stretched straight before her, knocking the toes of her combat boots together. It sounds like someone chucking nuts at a wall. "Pretty funny drawing in the guest book, Luke."

He tosses his chin in acknowledgment of her and then checks himself by pointing at her boots and mugging broadly. "You shine those yourself—just for the occasion?"

Janey's voice is ingenuous, sweet; she's pretty much puzzling over them for the first time herself. "I don't think they've ever been shined. I don't know, I just found them like this. I mean, they looked like this."

"Shiny," he says matter-of-factly.

"Not really—I mean these aren't really shiny, are they?"

Louise can't take it anymore, so she takes Luke's upper arm in her left hand, the "Stop tormenting Janey" grasp, though Janey is twenty-three and the combat boots evince more truth about her than the lace dress. When his mother drops her arm from his, her several gold bracelets slide back down, tamborining, a sound Luke could conjure with his eyes closed.

"Janey, your hair looks unbelievably normal—almost. I'm almost bored by it. Almost."

Luke and his mother have been lucky to find Janey, or Janey has been lucky to find them. He doesn't quite know, but she had darkened the doorway one evening perhaps seven years ago now—a petition for historical conservancy—and the next thing he knew, she was living at the house, companion to Louise day and night, both of them good together, funny, strangely inseparable. "It will come to an end," Louise tells him often enough, but he doesn't listen much to this comment, thinks it's a general pronouncement on the state of just about anything.

A young man in black robes stands at the front of the chapel now. His bright unfettered face is asking for the attention of the small group "willingly congregated here." He holds Glen and Naila's baby out to them, her small head in one of his hands and her bottom in the other. She is so miniature that her legs barely extend beyond his fingers, and he offers her to their care, the care of her parents' community. That's *classic*, Luke thinks, knowing his care is about the last care this baby's parents want. The presentation appears vaguely sacrificial to Luke and he begins to calculate just how willing he actually is to be here. Luke has enough children to care for, and this new one with her avid blue eyes calmly suffering the mosaic of faces murmuring their murmurings down upon her—aren't they phalanx enough? he protests. He could never willingly introduce such vulnerability into the world, and he doesn't want to be here being shunned at the same time as he's being called upon to accept more duty in this regard. Jesus, he thinks, Jesus, as they are instructed to take hands in a continuous and unbreakable circle around Glen and Naila and the baby, and then Luke looks beyond himself at the twenty or so people standing up and at the many hands beckoning and he traces with his eyes the long stretches of ivy and vine and flowers, how it all surrounds them, encircles them, ensnares them, he amends, ensnares. Louise is nudging him with her elbow, as if to say, HEY, get with the program. Stand up. But he doesn't like requests like this sprung upon him in social situations. He hasn't been asked—hasn't been allowed to think about it. He leans down to her because she wants his ear, and she whispers, "It's a christening, Luke. Give it a try," but he's not keen on this ritual, if that is what Louise is asking him to embrace. No shadows gloom her face, and he sees this difficulty is his alone. Her left hand is grasping his right, the long narrow fingers pulling him up, the heavily diamonded ring which had been his grandmother's hard against his knuckles. The chapel is so small, and made smaller by its vines and flowers, that the circle rounds from the front down through the pew where Louise and Luke and Janey have just risen. "This is Janey's new employer," Louise says, just when Luke is thinking this can't get much tighter, or more precious. "What do you think?"

He wants very much not to know what Louise has suddenly told him, but he doesn't have the energy to play dumb or surprised, though he is surprised, and surprised it's happened so soon. And he's angry. "You mean the florist, or whatever the hell you call this person Alice Samara—you mean Janey now works for her?"

Louise looks at him, her clear blue eyes taking him in; she knows her son, and she finds it interesting that her son knows this name, and the question plays for a moment across her eyes—How does he know the name Alice Samara?—but caution keeps her from asking. She can see he is struggling. "Yes, the florist," she says. Gravity leadens her voice.

"You don't call her a floral stylist?" Luke asks nastily, and his tone is the continuation of something Louise and he have argued about for months now, always in restaurants or in parked cars, away from the possibility that Janey might hear. "I am the psychiatrist," he had protested, "and I don't see the great unnaturalness of this relationship. I don't see what's wrong with having Janey in our lives. It's not as though you can't afford her."

"She needs to make her way in the world, Luke. She's talented and smart—I'm an old lady, and she honors me by being here. How you can imagine this as some sort of permanent position for her, I don't know. And anyway," his mother added, "*anyway*, two bad marriages and a dead child is not work that someone else should have to shoulder."

"What," he sputtered, his steak knife clattering down against the plate, "just what does that have to do with Janey?" But Luke knew for Louise that her past—theirs—had everything to do with Janey. "How can I ever pay Janey enough for making me happy in the way Sadie made me happy? How can I arrive at a conscionable salary for such a service?" And then not long ago, after weeks of Luke protesting, of Louise assuring him that Janey would always be in their lives, always, she had finally said, quietly, sitting in his car after dinner, "I can't love Janey like I loved Sadie, and if I could, then it might begin to be fair to Janey, but I can't. She's in contrast always, and a sorry comparison to Sadie . . . and this situation is cruel to her, and maybe even cruel to me."

Luke looks down now at his mother's face, sees how quickly his displeasure has clouded her brow, has slackened her mouth and cheeks. He doesn't want to have caused this, and he looks up to see Janey's two differently colored eyes on him. It will be okay, they are saying, Okay, we're all okay, Luke. And then his eyes are drawn elsewhere as his left hand is taken up briskly by Sheila.

"She's lucky to have you," he manages to say hoarsely to Janey. "Whoever this Alice Samara is, she's very, very lucky," and somehow the words are coming from his mouth more fluidly now, easily, and he knows there's something in this haven of flowers surrounding him that rivets him, calms him. "I want to meet her," he says quickly. "At least do that for me," and Janey turns her head to the side, a quizzical look, and sweet, and then laughs.

"Oh, I don't know about that, Doc. She's not all that keen on entanglements."

"Whom do you want to meet?" Sheila asks.

Luke pulls his hand from hers and makes a sweeping gesture of the chapel. "Whoever it is who did whatever this is," he says, looking at Janey, at her goofy, knowing smile. It makes him happy, and no, he doesn't want to think of her on earth instead of his sister; he doesn't want that, an exchange . . . and yet she is, too, and that is all all right, he thinks, Janey here now, and whole and well and smiling, but Luke hears his mother whispering, angry and sad, "Janey is not a replacement or a surrogate—instead, she's become something that allows my anger to mount further and further, to be rationalized. I find myself thinking if it had only been some other child who died, if it had only been Janey instead of Sadie—if only it were Janey who was dead." He can hear the anguish in his mother's voice, can hear her say, "Certainly your training prepares you to view that as fairly violent behavior to someone else!" But it isn't *behavior*; he argues with her now, even in his mind, "you could not have treated Janey better, or more kindly. You have thoughts occasionally, and so don't we all, but they don't dictate how you are to her." But now he can see all his arguments were useless, a waste of oxygen.

Glen and Naila's baby is being carried around the circle. Everyone is to reach out and touch her, to make their oath to her. Sheila is gazing down into the tiny face, seemingly at a loss for words, and then she says, "Hey, what can I say, I'm your aunt—I'll take you shopping." Luke thinks that right about now—if this baby has any self-respect—she should set to squalling.

And what the fuck do you want me to do here, Glen? Luke seethes, because now she is before him, this little one in her tiny white dress. She smiles from deep within her roses and chortles up at Luke, a far more animated response to him than to anyone else, and suddenly, Luke will take all of this, will accept whatever responsibilities he might have to this baby so much like Naila, her mother. He takes the baby for a minute completely into his hands, holds her against his chest—against his heart, he realizes—and then he hands her back, reluctantly, she as reluctant as he, her eyes casting back. For the first time today, he wonders what her names are, this new baby kicking her legs jauntily against his touch. She smelled like roses.

"You always were good with children . . . and maybe you still are." Louise laughs and pulls his hand up into her chest, just below her breasts. "My boy," she says, and Luke relaxes a little in her pride, the cold onyx button sharp against the back of his hand.

After the baby has passed from them down the pew, he asks, "When were you going to tell me about Janey? You pick today specially?"

But he realizes that Louise has told him before today, just not very overtly, has told him about Janey's interviews, about Janey being gone so much now. He realizes Louise has been calling him more recently, goading him into dinner. He wasn't paying attention, and he should have been. He'd canceled a date last Saturday because Louise had called, had said, "come to dinner," but then he'd used Louise as an excuse. "My mother's having a little catastrophe," he'd said to the woman, to yet another one he wasn't so much into as he was into having a date, making a reservation, going out on the town. Louise had saved him from feeling bad for this woman, for his use of her. "You have a lucky mother," she signed off with, and the woman had meant it, had been being kind, though Luke hadn't gone to Louise's, had instead gone to the club and smashed balls against the four tall walls so fiercely, the sharp vibrations made his wrist ragged and loose. And then the men's locker room mirror hadn't made it better afterward either, his too-bright face around the haggard eyes. Could he call the woman now, three hours past their original time, and say, Hey, I'm free now, how about at least a drink? He was marveling at himself, at going from canceling the evening, with no alternative future plan because he had no intention of ever calling her again, to calling her up and trying to salvage what was left of the night. Not only had he not kept Louise company, nor this tall young woman he'd met at a UCLA conference, a post-grad in clincial psychology, but he hadn't even suited himself particularly well, either. Certainly he hadn't paid enough attention to his mother to know she was telling him something about Janey, or trying to.

"You're coming with us to lunch, aren't you?" Louise asks now, but she senses the answer and smiles weakly. "Yes, okay, but call." He leans down and kisses her smooth cheek, and then turns to Sheila and gives her a great smooch on the lips, wondering as he does so why he is. People are moving from the chapel into mottled sunlight, passing Glen and Naila and touching the baby once more as they go. Lunch is close by, on campus, in a carved and paneled room preserved from a mansion demolished in the feckless eighties, and it's Louise who has gotten Glen and Naila this priviledge, and Louise who has seen to the catering and cake. She was the daughter of a state senator, her mother fragile and distracted, and she had taken over the many duties of entertaining and socializing. "Someone must be queen of taste," she'd always said, apologetically, and yet she knew so many people, and she knew how to do things and to do them well, and even though Luke does have two hours before he needs to be back in the office, he's not going to lunch; he's made that decision an hour ago. He hangs back and watches

Glen hold the door for his wife and child, and then the chapel is empty, darkened, and Luke sits down again, just to be here awhile, quietly, alone, enshrouded in vines and flowers. He can't quite believe he's managed to stay here unobserved, and it's a gift to him in this moment. He rises and walks to the front, to the font, and looks down into the shallow pool of water, where three white rose petals float. He pulls his fingers through the water and the petals stick and he holds them to his nose. They barely smell of roses. Her name is May, May Aisha. He dips his fingers again and the petals slide back into the water. He looks at the rose canes circling the font and sees now the fine green wire twisted carefully about the canes to make them stiff, and how one cane reaches all the way up and then hooks down across the lip of the font and that this one holds all of the others. I see, he says quietly, I see. He hunkers down and looks at the tightly rounded dome of green, green moss at the base of the font. He pulls it back, and beneath it sits a bundle of plastic water vials, into which all the ends of the canes lead. "Hide your mechanics," he once heard his mother instructing Janey. "Don't let them see your tricks." Samara—it can't be her real name, he thinks. It's part of a tree, or something, the seed, which he supposes is the fruit, too, but he doesn't remember all that much from the one botany class he ever took. "'It takes a superior mind to appreciate a plant,'" his mother quoted, "so for God's sake, take at least something botanical." Spinoza, Luke surmises, his mother was quoting someone like that.

Luke hears his next appointment in the anteroom just beyond his office, the unusual sound in his waiting room of a little girl's voice, that of Polly Markens, normal development till she reached the age of six years, two months, and then, as closely as he can tell, classical autistic behavior, unresponsive verbally and physically, an abhorrence of anyone touching her, echolalia, the use of the first-person pronoun suddenly absent from her speech, and in its place a fiercely interiorized affect. Because it is a little girl's voice, because it is Polly, he takes especial note. Autism is much more unusual in girls, though dissociative behavior is not, and to Luke there seems something *learned* in Polly's behavior, something being mimicked, enacted. What or whom she might be mimicking, he does not know, cannot glean from sessions with her parents or siblings. He is used to a complex and subtle originality in each of his patients, even when the individuality gets subsumed beneath a diagnostic label. Stan Mingis's non-responsiveness differs greatly from the manner in which Zeke does not respond, or from the lack of response typical of Henry Lutins, who is now fourteen years old and still barely speaks.

Polly, though, remains generalized, almost a stereotype of autism. She troubles him in great part because she fits a rubric too well—a rubric Luke has never actually seen organic in his nine years of practice. But six years of age is pretty late for autism to be diagnosed. He's been seeing her for six months and he still feels puzzled, duped really, as though she might be playing him for a fool. But you don't call the bluff of a six-year-old without anything to offer in return. No happy child manufactures isolation of this intensity for no good reason; it just doesn't happen. Then again, she might not be manufacturing anything.

He lets his hand drop from the telephone and swivels around in his chair. He'd been starting to call Janey, though what pretext he might use had stayed his hand. Could he actually ask her if she'd driven Louise home from the christening? His mother is a perfectly good driver at seventy, and who knew what plan they'd cooked up—they didn't need Luke to help with that! He realizes there are all sorts of questions to ask Janey: When did she start work with Alice Samara? What sort of medical coverage was there—*was* there medical coverage? When would she be at the house? But Luke isn't much interested in these specifics. He wants to meet Alice Samara; this he very much wants to do. Polly's file is lying in a basket on the credenza behind his desk. He doesn't open it, reciting to him-

self a file he has pored over, read and re-read, listening to the
tapes of her parents and of the brother and sisters, taking the
tapes with him in the car. He has Polly on B_6 and magnesium,
has sent her for allergy testing, an exhaustive neuro workup,
CTs; in fact, all four of the Markens children are as healthy as
they come.

He turns sharply back to his office and pushes the buzzer
affixed within the kneewell of his desk. Albertine's dark hand
gently moves Polly through the door and into his office and then
disappears. He can see Albertine's torso through the frosted
glass of the door.

Polly stands in precisely the same place Albertine has urged
her to with her hand. She has thick curly hair, which surrounds
her small head like a blond wig. She does not look left or right,
does not seem to focus on anything in front of her, either. Her
hands hang at her sides. "Why not come in, Polly. Sit down.
We'll have a talk."

"Why not come in, Polly. Sit down. We'll have a talk."

He has often, in moments of bemusement, thought that no
one is more careful with language than he is, as he spends most
of his days having it repeated back to him, and now, something
in the alteration of tone that Polly uses makes him hear his own
falseness. There seems every reason in Polly's world right now
not to enter this room, not to sit down and have a talk. He recognizes the threat, appreciates why she'd rather do almost anything but what he suggests. Here is an established office with a
gently prodding nurse within a huge edifice of a building, a
place merely by virtue of its architecture outfitted to menace
Polly down to size, to intimidate her into behaviors others
understand. Why the hell would she want to come in and sit
down and allow him to analyze any word of her own language,
her own choosing? Not a twitch of her cheek, not a word even
just starting to germinate within her mouth is safe from
scrutiny. Luke wonders why he feels this so strongly with Polly
before him? Why doesn't he have these raging empathies for
Stan, or Henry, or Zeke? He's not so used to treating little girls,
but something about Polly's behavior seems deeply, even pro-

foundly, justified. Something has gone down in her life; he feels sure of this. Maybe it was the whirlpool of too many changes at once: She had started kindergarten and was no longer at home, a place she seemed to like being. A baby brother arrived when she was four and a half, a battering ram of a child whom even Luke has observed with raised eyebrows. She now shares a bedroom with an older sister, when before she had had her own. A culminating tantrum had taken place the day her baby brother "rearranged" her desk and a table, where she had projects—a tiny loom, boxes of glass beads from India and Europe, and a collection of leaves and pods and seeds, items she gathered from the yard as carefully as a botanist, as assiduously as a bird building a nest.

"Polly, you used to have a room all your own," Luke says to her now, rising, not waiting for her to respond, "and Albertine and I thought that maybe you'd like to have that room again."

Polly speaks his words back to him. He doesn't listen as he crosses his long carpeted office to the door of the supply closet, but his words—"thought that maybe you'd like to have that room again"—hang woodenly in the air, effectless. What tremendous powers of refusal drain the word *maybe* of all its tension, its sense of possibility? He thinks that he'll throw the word back at her, see if he can't induce her appetite. He says, "The nurse and I thought that maybe you'd like to have a room again, one which you can visit every time you have an appointment, one which will be yours, here for you, all you own, that no one else will touch or disturb."

Polly repeats all he says.

He had thought to make a sign for the closet door, POLLY'S ROOM, but that seemed akin to the type of plasticized, self-conscious therapy that made intelligent people scoff and that went a long ways to legitimizing their rejections of "help." He had imagined Polly shaking her curly head before the door and then battening herself even further into isolation. He pulls the door open and the light comes on. The low table and chairs that Polly had had at home are now here, as is the small metal bead loom, and hundreds of various jars and vials, her own beads, her entire collection. At first, Luke had spent much time trying to figure out how to duplicate the table and chairs, how to re-create as closely as possible the trays of treasures, the old marcasite beads on the metal loom, the tiny Czechoslovakian glass globes her aunt had brought her from Eastern Europe. But if he removed Polly's table from her home, he wasn't sure what she would do in response, and yet it would have taken hours of roaming shops, "bead stores," Luke assumed they were called. He'd asked a woman he was dating at the time about just where such things were acquired, and she'd shown immense skepticism that a six-year-old child could weave beads. "Oh yes," Luke had said, "the designs are very intricate—I think they represent body parts—but no one else has done the weaving, believe me." There was something in the tone of his voice perhaps? The woman had looked away, and Luke could see in her smooth, lovely face the desire, a prayer really, for the children in her future to be normal, to be as unexceptional as possible, just so they were normal. She then picked up her napkin and blotted her mouth slowly and said, "There is a store on Main Street in Santa Monica; it's called Ritual Adornments. They will have almost anything you could possibly need for your patient." Their desserts came, and they took bites of each other's, bourbon tapioca and marjolaine crossing the table, spoon passing fork, but Luke sensed the date was over, that somehow he represented to her the possibility of a botched and difficult future. As he paid the valet for both cars, loading her into her sensible Subaru, she looked up at him and said, "There's another one; it's on Beverly, just east of Fairfax. Called Sweet Beads. That's a good store, too." Her car door closed between them and then caught a smear of light as she pulled from the parking lot into the busy swiftness of La Brea Boulevard. Not for her were Luke and the crazy, weird, impossible children he loved.

It had not occurred to Luke that Polly was extraordinarily coordinated, capable of motor skills and an attention to handwork that was exceptional. Then again, all autistic children were unlike other children, and most of them showed some extraordinary skill that others in their rage for normalcy, or uniformity—

he wasn't sure which—deemed beyond children of this age. Children in China, India, Guatemala—these children embroidered, wove, sewed, and this was called child labor, child abuse, and forced, it might be, certainly, but it was also evidence of ability at a much younger age than was *allowed*. He wondered who had given Polly the loom, who had taught her to string it. He knew from Jordan Markens that Polly practiced these activities on her own, worked quietly and happily—had never been forced. Finally, Luke had ventured to ask that Polly's table and collection be moved to his office, had nerved himself for puzzlement and a refusal, but his request registered only mild surprise on the Markenses' faces, and then Jordan Markens herself had said, "It can all fit in the car. I'll bring it tomorrow."

"Polly, come," he says. She turns on her heels and walks to Luke, and just the way she does this, not robotically, but quickly, almost snappily, makes him doubt her autism, or moreover doubt its origins as organic. Unless he just knows nothing after nine years of treating autism, her movements derive from personality.

She stands to the side of him now, not the side that will allow her access to the small room, but on the other side, her gaze boring a hole at the center of the door. She comes to his waist. He does not put his hand on her head or back, does not physically maneuver her around to the room's entrance. He hunkers down, holding on to the doorknob. "Have a look," he says, his arm stretched out between himself and Polly, and this is meant to be quite intentionally another obstacle to her seeing the interior of the room, to her entering. Can he get her to bristle? To move of her own will toward something she wants? He can smell her, and she smells like dry earth.

"Maybe you have some work to do," he says, and he realizes he's learned the word *maybe* from her, this word of inquiry now implacable as leg irons. He then allows a pale tincture of admonishment to color his words, though it's just that. "Come on," he says. He looks across at her small face, at the shrouded eyes beneath the overhang of blond curls. Four days ago, Polly had been so upset at the prospect of a haircut that she'd reached out and grabbed a rat-tail comb from a stylist and stabbed at herself in the chair. Luke hasn't admitted this to her parents, but the episode heartens him, its insistence, not only on not having a haircut but in attempting to feel her body active by struggling to cause it pain. If she can feel pain, she can know she is alive, a certainty principle that makes a tremendous amount of sense to Luke.

The telephone rings in the outer office, and as he listens— Is it Janey? His mother? Any of the parents of his patients?— Polly moves from his side and circles behind and then stands for a moment before the small room, a closet really. He cannot see what her eyes take in, but she enters the room, yanking the door shut after her, pulling him off balance because the door-knob gets so suddenly wrenched from his hand. He tumbles forward, and as he does so, a desperate adrenaline rises in him because the detonation of Polly's scream shatters his ears. They have not realized the light in the closet automatically goes off with the closing of the door, though of course, Jesus Christ, they knew it and didn't even think about it, hadn't, in the des-perate prospect of bringing inviolable space back to Polly's life, remembered that she needed light with which to see. So, danc-ing before Polly's eyes had just now been the vitrious blues, the faceted reds, the calm crystals—just for a magical feast of an instant before they took it away, those monolithic generators in the distance controlling her life, disappearing it, illusioning it, snapping it into darkness. It's all so fraught, Luke gasps to him-self, all so pitched and dire and unforgiving, but then Polly's scream, hollow now, screamed out, is an effect carried beyond its capacity to galvanize action. "Stop, Polly," he says. "Stop your screaming. Stop," he practically screams himself as he pulls the door wide open, and then Polly turns and looks him straight in the eye, eagles him into focus with such a raptorial glint that all becomes silent, even still.

He takes his time, lets this look have its full power, makes sure she sees her will is accomplished. "I'm sorry," he finally says, pushing the door back so it catches into place. "We only wanted you to have a room that was yours, with your projects in it. We forgot about the light."

She repeats only the last sentence back to him—"We forgot about the light"—but as she says these words, she pulls her tiny chair out and sits down. And then, so slowly that he doesn't see it at first, Polly pushes the other chair out from beneath the table with her foot. Luke looks down upon the painted seat of the little chair, a bright pink daisy with a yellow center. He thinks maybe Polly wants him to sit down. He also thinks that it's quite possible she never had the second chair at the table and doesn't want it there now. He wishes, as he often wishes, that he didn't work with such occult psychological circuitry. Or he wishes he had an intricately detailed map, or a guide, a Beatrice to lend him a hand. Here, in this room, in this closet, he wants a geography for Polly, a terrain beyond her own body that she recognizes as sovereign; if he treads there, he wants it to be by her invitation—*she* is Beatrice. He must wait to know if this moving of the chair is invitation or an attempt to re-create what she once had; and it's too soon to risk intrusion.

"Polly, I'm going to leave you to yourself," he says, moving back into the bigger empty space of his office. "No one will come in this room but you," he says, knowing that the minute Polly is picked up by her mother, he will open the door of this utility closet and study whatever order or pattern she has imposed here. He doesn't expect to learn much; probably there will be little to make a difference in her therapy. He's anxious, nonetheless, to see. But now he wants Polly to assure herself of the table's schema, to establish whatever intricate design constitutes for her physical cohesion. He assumes there will be a struggle when she has to leave, that she will not want to, or will quite reluctantly. He's surprised that Polly recovered so quickly from the lights shutting down. He thinks her more capable than most disturbed children of reasoning herself out of terror, which means she knows how to manufacture hope. This is unusual, or at least unusually early in someone with Polly's presentations. He knows Polly's IQ to be 145, which indeed is hope quantified, but of course not a guarantee. Her quick adjustment might also be due to the fact that she is here with Luke alone, and though he is threat enough, she knows he is not usually destructive of her physical world. Polly abides here more easily because of this, but as Luke strides across his office, he knows this is far removed from any world that Polly must learn to navigate, accommodate.

He has mounted a mirror set in such a way that he can observe Polly from a chair near his desk. It's not perfect, and he can't see everything, but it's enough of a view. He thinks of all the hours he spent watching Sadie, his sister, and there weren't any fancy mirrors, nor usually chairs, either, and he'd had plenty of resentment—and plenty of dope, too—to ease all of that. If he'd watched more carefully, he wonders now, if he'd paid any kind of attention whatsoever, might he have learned something important, or prevented what happened? "Stupey Lukey," she called him, but that had been only one name among dozens, and as he reaches for a tablet of paper from his desk, he sees her picture in its silver frame, the oddness of her distant eyes in her avid face. He pulls a chair from in front of his desk and positions it to face forward across the room and sits down. Now Polly's blond hair is tossing from side to side, an adamant jerk right, then left, mechanical, more like a toggle switch than something connected with tendons and vertebrae. Out of habit, he looks at his watch. He hears Polly's mother arrive in the anteroom, hears the quiet, deliberate exchange of words, the arrival of a parent a distinctly different audition than Albertine's pointed recognition of a child, her voice pitched higher, asking the questions adults always ask children, even autistic children.

Luke surmises that Polly knows her mother has arrived, that, in fact, the tossing is an attempt to ward off that knowledge, a defense against the inevitability of her removal from this office, her table, her body. Rising from his chair, Luke lumbers forward. He catches himself on the edge of his desk and leans there a moment. His legs spark and burn; the nerves dart down his calves, seize his thighs. He wonders how a culture ever came up with the idea of limbs being asleep, when rarely were limbs quite so maniacally alive! Polly's blond curls still toss; Jordan Markens is no doubt reading one of her many books on American politics; Albertine types out the next day's appointments—he can tell because there are no long stretches of sustained typing, no sentences, just short spurts of keyboard clatter. The nerve impulses subside and he walks across his office. His legs move gingerly at first and then comfortably, but replacing his own physical rigidity is now the image of Polly's hands grasping something within them so tightly that her knuckles appear like tiny dead racks of ribs. Probably she has beads in her hands, something that connects her to the table. He calls to her before he gets to the closet, "Hey, Polly, Miss Polly. I think it's a good idea to take some beads home with you, to keep them with you, remind you of your table here where you can work."

He continues, quietly, ceaselessly, to talk through her head tossing, not to stop it but, as gently as possible, to degrade the screen she is erecting against his inevitable encroachment. He wants to maintain for her as much of her own personal design of this moment as possible, as much of her singular will. He has not been able to bring himself to ask how Polly was restrained at the hairdresser's—hates the thought that in a few minutes he may have to restrain her himself, that she may try to hurt herself, may try almost anything to maintain her power over her own body.

"Polly, when you make yourself dizzy like that, isn't it hard to work at your table, hard to keep your eyes on what you're doing? Nobody will keep you from doing your beads here. We have to get that light fixed, but you're coming tomorrow. You can work then, and Monday." He looks at his watch. Three minutes. He actually doesn't know whether Polly's head toggling makes her dizzy; it may calm her, as Stan Mingis's spinning calms him. Albertine and Jordan Markens say something to each other, seem to be having a conversation, and it gives him an idea. There's too much pressure from the outside for Polly to leave without being forced. "Take your time, Polly. I'll be right over here at my desk."

Sadie stares out from her frame in half-light now. Luke runs his forefinger down her nose and then switches on the lamp. He sits down. He picks up his telephone. He thinks Sadie would not have been out of here for hours. He looks from his watch to the utility closet; the blond curls jump back and forth. Polly's been tossing for five minutes now. "Albertine," he says, "why don't you and Jordan come in, bring coffee or something, drinks, those fruit teas, like you're both going to stay for a while. Relaxed. I don't want you to seem like you're in a hurry. I'd like to see if we can't wait till Polly is ready to leave of her own accord."

Bring a bottle of wine from the fridge, he wants to say, bring a good white Burgundy, something not just dismally acceptable. Luke likes having things around that remind him of time, expertise, of process, care; nothing takes longer than waiting for a child to get better, and good things around him, which take time to create, to become what is valued, these help to assure him, and because he is most definitely not the only one who needs assuring, he would like to have a glass of good white Burgundy to hand to Jordan Markens, to watch the golden liquid moving toward her. From the day of vine planting, he would say, to what you're about to drink, this took at least five years. Longer. Let's allow Polly time.

He hangs up, knowing Albertine is not happy. She didn't sign on for socializing after work, and on a Friday, but when she and Jordan Markens come through the door, he's mis-read her tension on the line. He sees a small drama in her brown eyes. She has something she needs to tell him, and he realizes that if it were about a patient, she would probably just say it, speaking carefully so as not to use a name or much else to identify the person, perhaps putting a note inside a file and handing it to him. But she doesn't say anything, nor does she carry a file. He directs Jordan Markens to the couch, slides the low child's table over for the glasses and bottles Albertine does carry, and glances down the length of his office at Polly: eight minutes. He pulls the chair over a little closer to the couch for Albertine.

"Janey called," she says, sitting down.

"I'm sorry." Luke points, realizing he wants to have Polly in his sights and that the chair he's moved is too close to where he needs to be in order to see Polly. Albertine pulls herself out of the chair and moves to the couch. She's doing a masterful job of hiding her exasperation. "She wants you to call her back," Albertine says matter-of-factly. Luke nods. "I'll catch her later. Thank you. How are you, Mrs. Markens—Jordan?"

"Due home," Jordan Markens says in almost a whisper. He notices that she doesn't settle exactly, but leans her tall, reedy body somewhat stiffly against the cushions.

"It's all right," Luke assures her. "You can speak in a normal volume. We're not keeping anything from her."

"No, no, I don't. We don't."

"May I ask you," he says, keeping his eyes on Polly, "a little more about what happened at the hair salon the other day?" There's something of a small challenge in his words, something of a tiny gauntlet. Sometimes he can't help himself. It's his desire that his patients be handled well; it's his sense that in these moments of extremis patients are concertedly their most powerful and their most vulnerable . . . and vulnerable to therapy . . . and that parents are at their worst—and Jesus, who could blame them—though mostly, he knows, they are blamed and he a participant in this blame as much as he guards against that colossal stupidity on his part, the profession's part in its early days. "Who restrained Polly?" he asks. "How?"

Jordan Markens moves her back deeper against the cushions, her legs still straight out in front of her. She might be stretching, were it not tension she is working from her limbs. Her black slacks are tailored, elegant; she wears velvet mules. He reads the title of her book, *Why Americans Hate Politics*, and it's then that he sees the thicket of bright red scratches across both her hands; it's *then*, except it takes him a second to actually know what they are—because she's so fashionable, her hands could be a fine scarf, a touch of Japanese silk, plum blossoms against snow.

"How long did it take?" he asks.

The sadness they both share is not made better for the sharing, is too inevitably reflected back and forth and back and forth, the sadness for Luke that is Sadie—though Jordan probably doesn't know about Sadie—and the sadness that is Polly, a kind of somber, inarticulate ricochet of empathy that helps neither. Or maybe it helps them both; Luke doesn't know.

"Did you time her?" he asks, smiling. He wants to gentle her by bringing up the finite, the logistical, something she might have done, can do, can do in the future, an act specific and complete and unimposed upon by her personality, her intellect, her parenting, her desperate love.

She answers simply, a delicate exhaustion in her tone, "No, I'm sorry. I didn't."

The opening pop of a pressurized bottle lid sounds loudly in the room. Polly's tossing, which has been in his peripheral vision so steadily, now jerks to a stop. He turns his wrist to see his watch: eleven minutes. He likes Jordan Markens and wonders how she would test. So many behaviors are genetic, and more than a few are pathologized by a certain time and circumstance, rather than being just inherently the attributes of sickness. Luke wonders if Polly had been an only child, like her mother, if whether her present behaviors would have been provoked. Everyone has some sort of psychological arsenal, some hair-trigger ordnance, and it's almost always better left un-deployed.

Albertine, Jordan, and he touch glasses, a show of being relaxed. The glasses chime enthusiastically and he thinks, Thank God they didn't clunk woodenly, Thank God they didn't sound dead. He looks up at Polly's stationary curls in the mirror. He pulls a face of pleasant surprise at Albertine and Jordan. "Just a few minutes," he says softly to them both, putting down his glass. "Let's just see," and then they all hear it at once, the chair being slid across the linoleum floor, and looking, they see Polly pushing both the small chairs in under her table, her hands in fists, pushing at their top rails. She then turns in the narrow space of the closet and passes through the door. She does not close it. Luke assumes that grasped tightly in her fists are beads. He thinks quickly that he should have cataloged the table's contents more precisely but that in his hurry, his excitement to render the table safe from disturbance—and, by extension, her body safe—he had not thought to do so, just as he would not think to write down the parts of Polly's anatomy.

"Polly, it was lovely to see you today," he says to her. She stands directly before the office door, waiting patiently, resigned, docile, the exception to this mien in the balled tension of her hands.

Jordan Markens is already on her feet and Luke sees that she doesn't even take one more sip of her drink, that she was ready to depart as of ten minutes ago. Her sufferance bothers him, but he feels himself mean for even thinking the word *sufferance*; she has three other children and a husband who takes up all the oxygen. Luke thinks that probably even the children fight for oxygen in that house. Luke is immoderate, though, being immensely unfair, and he doesn't like to be this even in his mind; it's unconscionable for him to suggest that Stewart Markens is at fault for Polly's illness, for any part of it. But the guy so obviously takes what he needs, every bit, the house in full throttle for him—his high-powered lawyer's life. He's like a fetus, Luke thinks, the body supplying him constantly, assiduously, all needs met—the fetus completely unconscious of its treachery.

"How is Stewart?" he asks Jordan Markens before he begins the work of getting Polly to acknowledge that their session is over and that she has duties that she must perform, recognitions she must mark.

"Stewart?" Jordan says. "I'm sure he's fine."

It's an odd reply, and Luke lets her see he thinks it's odd.

"I mean, I haven't seen him all day," she says.

"No, of course not—I didn't assume you had." Luke continues to face her, to allow the full puzzlement of his face to sink in.

"I'm sorry. I just thought that you meant in this moment how was he."

It is interesting to Luke—actually fairly disappointing—that a form of social decorum that his field has found vastly important in helping children develop an ability for adaptation and adjustment is, in fact, something lacking in so many who would be considered—he would have to admit—healthy folk walking about. And it's not that Jordan Markens has just been outrageously rude; it's her tone, and the puzzling, alchemically puzzling, reconstitution of the question "How is Stewart?" into something confrontational, intrusive. What Luke is about to enact—to attempt to enact—is the recognition on Polly's part that he is not a piece of furniture, that the past hour has happened within a context, that she comes here for a reason, an important reason, and that words, and handshakes, recognize and respect these activities. That Luke has asked Polly's mother how her husband is and the answer was not only not forthcoming but polemical rigidifies his body. But as quickly as his anger has wired him up, he knows he must cut himself down from it, must indeed hunker down before Polly and reach out his hand and get her to shake it, entice her into saying good-bye.

"We'll fix that light, Polly," he says. "I'm sorry about that." He tells her she will come again tomorrow, that her schedule has been altered a bit so as to assure her of her room—her table's inviolability, its physical integrity, which, Luke surmises, is part and parcel of Polly's own sense of physical composure. He sees her clenched fists and doesn't think it wise to compel her to shake hands, though they've worked on this for months. "I think it pleases you that your table is here, doesn't it, Polly? That you may come here and work at it, may have your own little workroom? Tomorrow it will be just as you left it today. You needn't worry. Good-bye, Polly."

"Good-bye, Polly," she says woodenly.

"Good-bye, Doctor," he says, straightening his legs, rising up.

"Teeth," she says, "they are all teeth and will bite you."

"If I enter the room, Polly, is that what you're saying, that if I enter the room, I will be bitten by all those teeth?"

Polly smiles from beneath the blond overhang, her eyes glassed over and staring far beyond the door Luke is now pulling open. "This worked well," Luke murmurs to Jordan Markens. "I'm encouraged."

"Thank you," she says, holding the book to her chest and then fumbling one hand toward his, shaking it somewhat feebly, though not wanting it to be a feeble handshake and so not quite letting go, but re-collecting his hand into hers, strengthening her grasp momentarily, even affectionately, almost as though she does not want to let him go. "I'm sorry, thank you—"

"Hey." Luke smiles, the transfer of the parent to Albertine easy now, smooth, his hand on the telephone to call Janey as his office door closes, the number dialed as the outer door moans open, and Janey's voice on the line as the outer door closes, Albertine's dark face beyond the frosted pane, and then her double tap on the glass to say good-bye when she knows he is on the phone, and then again the outer door opening and closing, and then quiet.

"Not to worry, Luke, I got her home. She's perfectly fine to drive, though, as you well know—don'tcha! Since when have you worried about Geez Louise's driving?"

Janey's voice couldn't be admonishing if it tried, and she is trying, but Luke's not paying much attention to admonishments from Janey. "The two of you driving together is a hazard to us all," he says, wanting her to laugh, this youngun who turned up one day and made his mother's life a lot happier—his life, too. But now she has a job, or rather, another job, one outside his mother's house, the only house Janey had ever lived in, or at least that is what she had told them. Rooms, she and her mother had always lived in rooms—she did not use the word *apartment*—and then once in a basement with water running down the walls, that's what she said, "water just sheeting the walls." Doesn't that have to be fanciful? Luke had thought, hearing it at first, but the longer Janey had stayed, the longer she had talked and been with them and settled in, the more Luke believed her, saw that what she had managed to grow up within was probably worse than she described. "Family? Sure there was family," Janey said, "but why would I seek out the people who threw my mother out of the house pregnant with me—they sure as hell don't want anything to do with a bastard, and who knows who my father is, probably my grandfather," Janey added, rolling her eyes. "God knows, and God's a master of the secret, believe me." But so in a way was Janey, too, and it had taken Louise almost a year to find out if Janey's mother was alive, or near, or just what had happened? "I like houses," Janey said. "I suppose that's kind of simple, isn't it, liking houses because I never lived in one? But that's why I volunteered to walk petitions around for historical preservation. I got to see some beautiful homes from standing on the stoop, biding my time, talking until they invited me in." How Janey's sunny disposition had ever come about, let alone survived, was a mystery to Luke and his mother, but it had gotten her through many a door, including and most particularly his mother's. "Oh, she's dead," Janey had answered simply one morning, perhaps surprised anyone would want to know. "I have her with me," she added. "My mother's ashes. They're upstairs — I hope that's all right."

"Come on, Luke," she says now. "Come on."

"Come on what?"

"It's no big deal, and Louise is really happy about it. I think she was getting sick of me always being there anyway."

This last is not true, but Janey is no fool, either, and she's picking something up.

"That's not it, Janey. My mother adores you. Do you have medical coverage? Is this full-time? I mean, who is she, your employer? How big a business is this?"

"I've got all that. Do you know she's never taken on an assistant who actually helps with the flowers—I mean, she has guys who carry stuff, that sort of thing, and drivers, but up to now she has done all the work alone. Isn't that quite amazing?"

"Janey, I'd like to meet her, as I said at the christening. What does she look like anyway?"

"What does she look like?" Janey repeats his question, a kind of mock incredulity inflecting her words. "What does that have to do with anything? Luke, look, I think she's kind of reclusive. Plus, she works a lot."

"I think I'm not surprised to hear that, after seeing the chapel today."

"Amazing, huh?"

"You didn't help with it, then?" he asks, knowing the answer. He looks down at the tablet of paper on his desk and reminds himself to make notes on Polly before he leaves this evening. Speaking of working a lot, he thinks, worn-out, he had better start to work on guidelines for L.A. County Unified. He can't decide whether the idea of mainstreaming children with autism into the public schools is good for anything but getting moneys from the government. He knows the encapsulation of his patients is not broken down by proximity to others, and he fears mainstreaming may actually be a very bad idea. He'd better order food up, he realizes, he'd better start to devise the questionnaire for compiling data—God knows when he'll get home tonight.

"I start on Monday," Janey says, happy surprise in her voice, "because I guess in the flower business Mondays are really slow."

"You'll do that for me, set up a meeting, yes?" Luke asks.

Janey's response comes slowly, thoughtfully, "I don't think she dates."

As he hears these words, he sees the small dark-haired woman in a white shirt entering the chapel he had just left. She carried a black plastic bag as big as she was, and it had billowed out behind her and about her ankles, and then two young men in black T-shirts and jeans had followed her in, both carrying black plastic bags, too. He felt very sure the woman had been Alice Samara.

"What do you mean, you don't think she dates, and how would you know such a thing anyway?"

"Gossip," Janey says, her voice quiet over the phone. She is not a person who likes to tell tales on others. "That's all. I just heard a few stories."

"Seems I'm the last to know anything about this person who—"

"That's how I got the job, someone who knew someone who knew your mother. You don't want me to move out, do you, Luke?"

He is a little stunned by this question, and wants to tell Janey something that will finally relax her with respect to her presence in their family—she is family and Louise would suffer hugely if Janey left completely. Louise had said, "I want her to have something, Luke, at least enough for a down payment on a house—or if she ever wanted to finish high school and go to college. Don't you think that's a good idea?" And he had thought it a good idea, and the lawyer had been called, but he can't tell Janey anything of this nature, as he knows she will perceive it as some kind of restraint, or debt. Somewhere along Janey's short way, she had picked up very old school values. "Janey, where do you get such ideas? Move out. Christ almighty. There's not enough room for you there?"

Janey laughs a little on the line, and Luke wants to reach out through the wires and shake her. Seven, maybe eight years she has lived on Elmwood Drive with Geez Louise, as she calls his mother, and Louise has wanted Janey to emerge in some way, to seek a world for herself, but she hasn't wanted Janey to leave. Ever.

"Get me an appointment with Alice Samara," Luke now says.

"But it's okay, yes?" Janey asks. "It's okay that I'm going to be working with her?"

Luke doesn't immediately answer. Where should he order food from for dinner, he wonders? Can he survive another deli meal? "Sure," he says finally, because what else is he going to say? What else can he say?

Luke draws the razor down his cheek slowly. He savors the frisson, the blade against nerve endings, follicles, the added tension of a cheekbone, a chin, the razor sliding over neck and tautness and tendons, but then, he has not cut himself, and this is always a small amazement to him, a reprieve, and so he begins again, just beneath his temple, his eyes tracking the path of the razor in the mirror.

He thinks about her now, that he will meet Alice Samara today, at last, downtown, where her business is, where she works, where Janey works. After Stan Mingis's appointment at nine, he has two hours, some scribbled directions, a vague sense of whereabouts: a grimy warehouse district alchemically now chic, and Alice Samara somewhere there among the bricks and girders—among, he presumes, flowers, foliage, some densely created cloister. He has waited too long to do this, to find this person, to determine if what he fathomed some months ago is correct . . . or merely eccentric professional surmise. He thinks again about the first time he saw her work, how it startled him, not because her flowers were beautiful or unusually profuse or decadent, but because they were to him strange and edgy and uncanny, nothing that flowers, their arrangements, had ever been, and a little crazy, too, and creepy, *creepy little monkey*, he quotes absently, getting ready for Stan, lines from *The Lion King* weaving their way in and out of his thoughts. Who hires work like Alice Samara's to be done? he'd thought while sitting in the chapel that morning, except in that first instance, the christening, he'd known the people very well, Glen and Naila, and all of them doctors, though still his question remained unanswered, or maybe not who, but why?

He hears the telephone ring in the den, once, and then the service picking up. He looks out the bathroom door to the clock on his dresser: 6:49. Someone trying to hold on for 7:00 A.M., even 8:00 A.M., but who finally can't. He'll call in when he finishes shaving. His arm aches from racketball last night, an oddly desultory game he'd picked up with someone he'd seen only once or twice at his club. He thinks the guy has found out somehow that he's a psychiatrist. Off the clock, Luke thinks, that's my time, but the guy kept bouncing the ball, long pauses before serving, chatty questions that Luke had answered with a clipped firmness of speech that was—thank God—the prerogative of male exchange. A telephone sounds again, this time his cellular from the closet. That is probably Albertine telling him whom the call just before was from. She often started picking up calls from her house, before she was even due at the office. He wishes, in a way, that she'd not do that. He doesn't pay for a monopoly on her time. He'd set her up with cellulars, one for the office and a personal one, but he hadn't realized just how assiduous she would be. She has her own life away from these kids he treats, a son in the Coast Guard, a husband, but Luke should have known, kicks himself for not remembering how Albertine is.

"You ever notice," she'd said to him a few day ago, "you ever notice that lots of case studies claim an autistic's told 'fantastic stories,' but then those stories aren't there in the profile? Why is that? You'd think that would be very important, would contain all sorts of insights and clues. Plus, it just would make much better reading!"

Luke wipes his face down, hearing Albertine's voice in his mind, expecting that same voice as he pushes on the cellular he's retrieved from his closet. Instead, there's a weird silence on the line and then a shrill jangling clatter, as though someone has just dropped a whole rack of pots. Sadie, he thinks, all wrong numbers are Sadie, all irretrievable transmissions, all crossed wires—all Sadie, his sister, dead twenty-one years now. Good morning, he says to her, good morning, Sadie.

"I'm a doctor, Stan, your doctor—" Luke says, rising from his chair as Stan comes through the door, Stan already talking, moving his straight blond hair from side to side.

"Raymond Shaw's the kindest, bravest, warmest, most wonderful human being I've ever known in my life," Stan shouts.

"No, Stan, you don't know a person named Raymond Shaw. He's a character in a movie, in a novel first," Luke amends, because that is precisely the type of detail linguistically sophisticated children often insist upon, "a novel by Richard Condon titled *The Manchurian Candidate*."

"I'm merely commenting on the differences in your royal managerial approaches," Stan states matter-of-factly, the green pencil at rest, held perfectly still mid-air.

"Do I scare you, Stan? Like Scar in *The Lion King*? The mean uncle? Do I scare you?"

"It means no worries for the rest of your days."

"What does, Stan? What means no worries for the rest of your days?" Luke knows that if Stan replies "Hakuna Matata," he will have progressed far beyond any reasonable prognosis.

"Raymond Shaw's the kindest, bravest, warmest, most wonderful human being I've ever known in my life."

"Stan, do you feel that we've prepared a way for you to act or respond and that you must abide by that?" Luke asks this as he moves from behind his desk to the new drafting table where Stan draws. Luke folds and bends and tucks his long legs till he sits on the floor at the front of the table. Were Stan to look at him, he'd have to peer downward, but also, Luke knows, were Stan to look at him, something difficult would be about to happen. "Do you feel we control your responses, that there's a script that we've written?"

"Raymond Shaw's the warmest, bravest, kindest, most wonderful human being I've ever known in my life," Stan says quietly.

Luke laughs and pulls his back up a bit so that he's sitting straighter. "You've changed some words around, haven't you, old man?"

"They were killed instantly by a high mortar shell."

"Nah, Stan, stop it. Answer me. You moved the superlatives around, didn't you? 'Kindest, bravest, warmest.' You haven't done that before."

Stan reaches down and peels a page back on the tablet, holding it up so that Luke's face is blocked from Stan's sight. Luke speaks through the paper. "You want me not to be here, to disappear." Luke pauses, lets his spine slump again, leans back on one hand. Stan holds the paper very still, a tiny suspended screen, behind which he is completely obscured. "Hey, Stan," Luke says, "Why don't you ever write words down? Why do you always draw in the air when you're here? I know you can write your letters, words, sentences—you're the smartest kid I know." And you can't draw for shit, Luke thinks to himself, knowing Stan was treated for a year by someone who believed the key to autistic children was through their drawing, an approach which would be—*is*—fine for a certain type of autism, which Stan does not happen to suffer from. But breaking Stan of this performance is perilous because in one huge sense it's excellent that Stan has learned to do something in response to a situation not of his own making, and something that he thinks pleases authority; it's absurd when Stan enacts something undecipherable, diagnostically useless.

Stan rips the sheet of paper from the tablet now and lets it drop rather dramatically from his fingers. It flutters, hesitating, side-winding one way and then the other, and then settles flat. "You know that my entire life is devoted to helping you, helping my two boys," Stan says.

Luke starts to break out laughing and then holds it in, though just a little. Stan is autistic, no doubt about it; he is also funny as hell, intentionally. Luke knows he is, knows Stan knows he knows, and though Luke doesn't exactly want to encourage his speaking in lines only from *The Lion King* and *The Manchurian Candidate*, Stan's command of their comedic possibility is very funny. And very sophisticated. "That's the mother right? That's Raymond Shaw's mother who says that in *The Manchurian Candidate*," Luke says, "and one of those boys just happens to be a United States senator, right, Stan?"

Luke has observed many times that Stan enjoys the physical effect of humor on the faces of others, that Stan likes *seeing* people laugh. What muddles Luke is the issue of how psychologically perceptive one usually must be to have a sense of humor, to understand how to provoke laughter with language. The autistic who throws a vase on the floor because he enjoys the highly expressive look of anger on his mother's face has not had to master anything particularly intricate psychologically or linguistically; he's just tossed a vase. But what must Stan understand to provoke the physical expression of laughter that he seems to so enjoy—to provoke this with an intricate configuration of language?

Stan looks out over Luke's head, his huge dark eyes not focused, though not glazed, either. Luke would love to touch Stan, to hold him with all the affection he has for him, that language of acceptance that only the body speaks well, that only the body, its warmth, accents properly. He's sure that even an attempted bear hug, let alone one that actually achieved contact, would send Stan into furious dervishing. Sadie had been the same way, untouchable, explosive even if someone just grazed her shoulder. So Luke continues to talk, to wheedle out of Stan just how he is putting this script together. "Okay, so," Luke says, "the senator wants to cash in on Raymond Shaw, his step-son, being a decorated war hero; he wants this link with heroism to help with his re-election, right? Stan? You listening? You think your coming here helps me just as much as it's supposed to help you, right, Stan? I need you as much as you need me, that basically I'm campaigning here?"

"He's tall." Janey will have said that first, or possibly, "He's a doctor, a psychiatrist." Janey's capable of describing him to Alice Samara in any number of fanciful ways. He doesn't suppose—or even much hope—she waxed toward words like *handsome* or *intelligent*, a little sweetness and light on the subject of himself and why he's coming. "Knows a little something about wine. Reads a book occasionally." He grumbles, thinking Janey might have said, "He likes seeing his mother, the woman I used to work for—the woman I live with." Heaven save him if she has, though Janey's used the tag for years—"Mama's boy."

Luke glances across at Janey's runic directions lying on the passenger seat. She's used a wide-nibbed pen filled with fuchsia ink, and even if there's an architectural interest in the letters, and even if he knows Janey's twenty-three, the color splashed here and there across the page is pure adolescent girl. It's taken him several weeks to get these directions, and then a few more weeks to find a morning arrangeable enough to have time to make the trek. He's curious about why Janey's been so squirrelly about this. She cares for him, would probably do just about anything for him or his mother, and yet he's had to practically drop to his knees for this appointment. But then again, what is it exactly? It's not really an appointment.

He just wants to meet her, Janey's boss, this Alice Samara, legendary for her refusal to have a staff, legendary for the prices that accompany her creations, and now Janey is the only person who has ever worked with her. He just wants to watch her for a few moments, to see her work, to watch her hands. But Janey might as well be his little sister, her suspicions run so deeply. She thinks he not only wants to ravish her boss but also to check up on her, to check for his mother, who worries about Janey like a daughter. It's the district the studio's in, one inscrutable warehouse after another just off the Santa Monica Freeway, and downtown. If Janey—if anyone— were to scream for help, God knows what would scurry from the recesses, and God knows what their intentions would be. Louise worries as anybody might worry, and Luke is happy to give a fortifications report, but he's here for other reasons, too, ones Janey would not go near even if he tried to explain them, professional reasons. "Save your mumbo jumbo for your patients," she would say. "Don't pathologize the entire effing world."

Luke exits at Alameda, downshifting from fifth into fourth, then third, the car circling smoothly down under the freeway into the grubby darkness. The walls of the ramp are striped with tire marks and he wonders how they got there. Did people come off the freeway so fast that they lost control, their vehicles skidding up along the walls? Or were these motorcycle stunts? A confetti of glass glistens along the other shoulder, the one not banked, which confuses him. Was the glass swept there after an accident, or maybe, because there seems to be a rather serious amount of it, was it dumped there? He's not surprised artists find areas like this in which to be interested, in which to work—there is always the suggestion of event and narrative, of

56 · MICHELLE LATIOLAIS

work being done toward something, against something, and at once there's an elemental quality, the raw materials of civilization. It's all possibility and at once the disastrous result of possibility. He likes it, and he doesn't.

Under the freeway it is dark, and Luke sees nothing for an instant before the hot, grimy glare of a downtown Los Angeles morning blinds him momentarily. Then there is a filling station of no major gasoline brand, willfully derelict, one that might have been lifted straight out of a thirties crime novel. A dog runs a slalom course between the pumps, barking. Luke looks down at Janey's map, the geometric lines feathered periodically, directing him down an alley and then through a gauntlet of electronic gates to a small warehouse set behind another. Janey has given him a mysterious white card, which he dutifully feeds to each blinking aperture as it presents itself. All this security, and yet he still thinks that if his car's intact after he gets out of this place, he'll owe the Big Guy. Christ. But then again, maybe he'd sacrifice the car. Maybe. It's been so obsessional, his wanting to meet her—he shouldn't have bought her book, because the pictures had fueled him, had galvanized his attention and interest.

He kills the ignition, pushes the stick shift into reverse, and lets the clutch out. He's still unsure what to think of her flowers, whether he, as a man, *is* to think of them, or whether they are something only women talk about, exclaim over. Gay men? He resents all of these classifications, cannot curb his interest in what Alice Samara makes in the world, or makes *of* the world, he emphasizes, because the chapel on the USC campus was odd to begin with, not particularly pretty or serene, but substantially moody, dark, cool. Its warren-like smallness gave off—even before she decorated it—the suggestion of fairy tales, of animals and a forest, brooding, wild places where children were abandoned or rescued, where children ate berries to survive or imperiled their lives further by trusting witches. But Samara had merely intensified this suggestiveness, he thinks, by working vines in and around and through the pews, along the stone floors—an unnerving web, of cloister? of peril?—but somehow all of the vines not only led to but blossomed at the baptismal font, blossomed into the baby's gown, into the roses around her face and across her tiny kicking feet.

"What's she look like?" he'd asked Janey again at dinner several weeks back. "Give me a description," but Janey snickered and tossed her violet hair. "Okay," he said, trying another tack, "then tell me, is she married?"

"Oh Luke Luke Luke, not for you"—she sighed, waggling the salt shaker at him—"not for you."

He gurrumps even now. A woman who dyes her hair purple cannot possibly have a keen sense of sexual attractiveness. He throws his eyes at himself in the rearview mirror and decides purple hair or no, she's probably right, but he looks okay, rested at least, his hair not too recently cut. He doesn't appear too much like a professional man with every nerve ending cauterized because, God knows, if they weren't, who would live like this! But he doesn't look dickless in that way that totally dickhead professional men look. And he doesn't look like a total bum, either, doesn't look like he has his dick in his hand. He wonders how many times he can use the word *dick* in the course of getting himself from his car into the front of this industrial building? Dick, he thinks, where the hell did that come from? *Richard?* And because he's a psychiatrist, because he does this for a profession, he watches himself from some distance riffing on dicks and dickless wonders, and the entire time he feels his stomach frisking about like a fucking prawn.

Janey barely acknowledges him as she answers the door and leads him past several glass-fronted walk-ins and through a maze of buckets filled with flowers to what looks to be an elevator. "Don't waste her time," she says, swinging open a small metal box and pushing a black button, which rings a tocsin somewhere deep within the building. Her hair is no longer purple, but in the dimness he cannot make out exactly what color it is now, nor how it's standing up around her head like quills. "She doesn't know you're coming," Janey says, turning to face him, no small amount of exasperation in her voice. "And don't forget, I've got some seeds for Louise. I told her you'd bring them to her, because she wants to plant them this weekend, and I have to be in Malibu for a couple of days—a really huge wedding."

"What do you mean, she doesn't know I'm coming?" he asks. "Don't I have an appointment?"

"For what, Luke? An appointment for what? Huh? What was I supposed to tell her? I have this bach guy in my life, he's like a brother, sort of, and he jerks off to your flowers, and I just thought maybe you'd like to meet him?"

Luke doesn't exactly hate Janey right now, but he's not sure why he's suddenly on a par with some punk in a baseball cap? Why can't he just pay Alice Samara a visit and be received? Maybe he should have thought to come up with some order, but for what? He didn't tend to throw a lot of parties—any, for that matter—nor were there occasions in his life big enough to merit flowers, let alone a consultation about them. He'd placed orders with her before—flowers to be sent his mother, to Albertine—but all that entailed was a call to Janey.

"Couldn't you have said that I thought her work deserved some study? That I was a psychi—"

"Okay, let me rephrase. I have this guy in my life, he's like a brother, and he jerks off to your flowers *in his sphygmo-manometer*, and I just thought maybe you'd like to meet him?"

Luke laughs in spite of himself. "Christ, where'd you learn that word? Anyway, I don't use one anymore."

"Lovely, I'm sure."

"Janey," Luke says, "calm down."

Rising precariously in the freight elevator, Luke thinks good humoredly, This is a shaky start. Steel floor joists stripe past, then concrete subflooring, sunlight and a huge empty space—except for a desiccated pigeon by an iron column—steel joists again, more concrete subflooring, a room of mottled light and naked mannequins, and rising still, past another floor, this one covered in wooden pallets, upon which rest large canvases all turned to the wall. Toward the fifth floor, the lift starts to slow, then heaves and summits. Luke's stomach scrambles midair, bungies to his knees, and returns to his chest cavity only after what seems a very long time. Jesus, he thinks, don't throw up.

He rolls the rattling grille back and steps off the spongy lift. Across the vast empty floor of the loft, and at a point arbitrarily chosen, it seems, not mid-room, not cornered, not stationed near an iron column, she stands, bowered beneath several *Ficus benjamina*, one small black-heeled foot resting upon a stool rung. As he nears the area set off with the huge pots of ficus, he can see that her worktable horseshoes around her and that her hands weave a vine of sweet peas, a vine that now drapes off the table and travels for several yards. How does she keep them alive, fresh-looking? There are no water vials in sight. He wonders this as she picks up a spray bottle and mists the entire length of the garland, walking out into the loft, spritzing, spritzing, then walking back. She does not look over, and he realizes that she does not know he stands there. It smells lovely. He says "sweet pea" by way of identification, by way of introduction, "Sweet pea" just after the spritzing sounds die. These are sweet pea, aren't they? the intonation of his voice queries, but the face that turns to him has heard differently, has heard him call her "Sweet Pea," his voice asking, beckoning, "Is that you, sweet pea?"

He says nothing to disturb whatever chance or hope his words have presented to her. He'll not disturb the distant light brightening, warming her cheeks, enlivening her eyes. Not quickly, though not particularly slowly, she realizes what he's said, how he's meant it, that he's not called her "sweet pea," that he's merely been saying what the flowers are. "Yes," she says finally. "Yes, sweet peas, lots of sweet peas." She laughs, throwing her arms out by way of presentation. "And how the hell did you get up here?" she then demands, her gears deftly shifting, her voice now driving hard.

"I said I wanted to meet you. Janey's a—Janey used to work for my mother, before you hired her away. She still lives with— I'm Luke."

Alice Samara gazes at him, the spray bottle still held aloft in her hand, the other hand tucked to her stomach, the thumb tightly grasped within the fingers. "Luke what?"

"You always do that with your hand?" he asks, pointing.

"It's genetic," she says quickly, setting the spray bottle down, both hands flying back to weave the last sweet pea blossoms into the end of the garland. He thinks her hands move like fidgety birds atop a bush.

"Maybe," he says. "Maybe genetic."

"May I help you with something?" she says ironically. "With flowers perhaps? Someone agree to marry you, Luke with no last name?"

Now that he stands closer to her, he can see that she is small, really, and that out of her heels, she will reach just to his shoulders, not even. She wears slim black pants, black heels with no stockings, and a white sleeveless shirt open two buttons' worth to reveal the camber of her breasts. He has always loved that straight dramatic drop from a woman's neck and throat across the clavicle to the breasts just beginning to rise. Her skin is pale, overcast, and he wants to reach through it to touch her, to feel the small bones move beneath his palms, to run his fingers along those bones, their lengths, their shortnesses, to pull those bones into himself. Why he is so instantly on the inside of her, he does not know, but he is—is past the skin and dark eyes and small open face.

"That's right, isn't it?" he manages to say. "Grooms usually do flowers?"

"If you mean, pay for them, yes—grooms rarely *do* anything at all." She absently buttons and unbuttons the neck of her shirt.

"Hmm," he murmurs, not very amused, "no, I'm not getting married." She walks out from her horseshoe table and returns with a large plastic-lined carton. She sprays down the insides with water and then begins to coil the garland carefully into the box.

"Where's that going?" he asks.

"You wouldn't believe it if I told you."

"Probably I would. I'm a doctor—doctors know the weirdest stories."

"You're not a doctor for the Industry?"

"No," he says, laughing, "I'm a psychiatrist for children."

She leans down and pulls a receiver from a phone cradle that hangs on one of the legs of the table. "Janey, you want to come get Miss Peaseblossom's boa?" she says, fluting the words. Janey and she laugh at something, and then she says, "I know, I know, it's like doing business with people in their terrible twos. But phone them and tell them they've got only a few hours— maybe not even." She pauses again, listening, her gaze beaded on some distant point beyond the warehouse window. He tries to determine what she sees, what she is focused on so intently, but brick walls, large industrial windows flashing with sunlight, a scrawl of black graffito are all he can gather. "No," she says emphatically into the receiver, "they're not going to hold. Remind them." She drops her gaze to the garland, half of which is still draped across the table. "Yes, I know they know, but they work in a very different medium—theirs doesn't wilt." She switches the receiver to her other ear and then walks out from the table and pulls a smaller bucket of white sweet peas from among the larger buckets of purples and pinks and mauves. The coiled telephone cord moves across the table and he sees that there are leaves and small twigs and blossoms all furled within the cord, sticking out here and there, a kind of garland all its own. He thinks there might be days, even weeks, of floristing gathered within this cord, and then Alice is stretching the cord out several yards across the loft and leaves and petals are showering down onto the wooden boards, and then she pulls a green garden hose back across the floor to her table. "They're fucking lucky I made the garland in the first place," she says into the receiver, and then tosses it onto the table, where the cord, in constricting, gathers up a new supply of leaves and flowers. *Fucking lucky*, he repeats to himself, surprised a little that she seems tough, tough-minded. What was he expecting, a harp recital? Some apparitional creature? The goddess of spring? Actually, she's a lot smaller than he expected her to be. She's compact, charged. It's not the way her work is, and then he thinks better of that equation. Frank Lloyd Wright built some of the tallest buildings in the world in his time and yet he was practically a grease spot.

"Who gets the job of cleaning that?" he asks, pointing at the telephone cord slithering, gathering itself across the table. "Want me to hang this up?"

"Not really," she says. "What may I do for you?"

"You did a christening that I attended," he begins, remaining where he stands, anchoring himself almost; wants to get this right, he wants her to understand he sees something in her work. "It was particularly . . . I don't know, I mean I do know, particularly . . . I wanted to meet the person who thought to sew real sweetheart roses onto a christening gown."

"In your line of work, do you attend a lot of christenings?" she asks seriously. "Do you work with children, or with babies?"

"No," he says, "I don't attend many christenings, but you know, this baby seemed wrapped in flowers, roses at her feet and around her head and all around the baptismal font. I mean, I said to myself, Who is this person swaddling a child in leaves and petals—who is she?"

The hose has a valve at its nozzle and Luke watches her slowly turn it. He watches the water start to fill a low galvanized tub. She does not say anything, the green hose reaching out in its huge circle behind her.

"I read a book once, about Hiroshima," he continues. "I think we all read it in high school, by John Hersey, and there was this detail in the book, which I guess was true, is true, about how after the bomb people ran and hid themselves in trees and bushes and wouldn't come out for days, weeks even, living in the trees."

She is unscrewing the tops off several spray bottles and setting them along the side of her worktable, their filler tubes pointing out into the air like strange, singular antennae. She holds the bottles submerged in the tub two at a time until they fill. They begin to line the edge of her table and he wants to be doing something other than standing there, chattering; he wants to pick up the praying mantis tops of the bottles and screw them back on, or at least replace the receiver in its cradle. He wants to do something that helps her work; he can see, though, that one does not presume.

Finally she says, setting the last two bottles on the worktable, "It's a very interesting connection—I mean if that's what you're making, a connection." But she does not encourage him with any further recognition or identification of what he has just touched upon.

"I work with autistic children," he says. "High-functioning, maybe not autistic sometimes, maybe severe neurological problems that cause dissociative behavior—they're all different." He watches her methodically twist the top onto each spray bottle, top after top, till they are lined up once again, their heads all facing in one direction, a continuous and exact series.

Alice gazes out the window again. "You said 'she.' You said 'Who is this person swaddling a child in leaves and petals—who is *she*?' How did you know that it was a she?"

Of course, he had been told her name shortly upon first seeing the chapel, but he thinks to himself that definitely there's some bias here, too, some inherent surmise on his part. He supposes his bias has mythological foundations, Moses' mother making him an ark of bulrushes, Diana turning into a laurel tree, and of course sexually it appeals—he's fallen in love with her work, so he wants her to be a woman, available. "I don't know how I knew," he says. "Perhaps the work just had a gendered appeal to me. Then, of course, I was told your name, and then I saw your book, and that masterful picture of your back." He laughs. "And were there any doubt at that point, the dust jacket uses the feminine pronoun."

"Yes," she says absently, "of course, the book—I always forget about the book. It's strangely permanent. I'm not used to the flowers being permanent—I don't like that the book doesn't wilt and fade and die back."

We're not talking about flowers, he wants to say to her; we're talking about you. Instead, he asks, "But don't you have books of designs for customers, guides of sorts?" He can see that she is not inclined to answer, that perhaps she has not even heard the question. Her arms are filled with spray bottles and she walks around into her horseshoe and then lines the bottles up on the shelf beneath her table, their heads once again all pointing in one direction, their bases spaced out evenly. She rises up and reaches for the telephone receiver and returns it to the cradle. A small wooden hand broom hangs to the side of the telephone and she uses it to brush stems and petals from the table. She brushes all in one direction, away from the tub of water, and when she's finished, she hangs the broom back onto its hook. He can see that she barely remembers he stands there, near her, that if he does not somehow stay her attention with a spoken sentence, even an arm held out to her, that she will further enfold herself, till the chance is lost and a spoken word, an arm, will startle her.

"May I take you out?" he asks. "I can't claim that it's always the most relaxed experience dining with a doctor. With my patients, I'm pretty much always on call, but I'd like to take you out. To dinner," he adds. "A place you'd like."

At the head of her table sits a large, flat robin's egg blue box. She pulls it toward her and lifts off the lid. "Oh," she says as she slides a newly polished silver salver from its felt cover, which is the same shade of turquoise as the box. He thinks there is something about the salver that surprises or puzzles her, that perhaps she has asked for a different one, one smaller or bigger. "Not what you wanted?" he asks her. "The tray?"

She doesn't look up from the silver salver, onto which she now has stuck four small pieces of green putty. She secures the stem of a huge ivy leaf into each piece of putty so there appears a cross of leaves against the blue silver. "Oh," she says again, even more distractedly, showing no sign that she has heard him, and then she walks with a small circle of green florist's foam to the tub of water from which she has filled her spray bottles. As she holds the oasis on the surface of the water, letting the foam absorb slowly, she looks up at him, her dark hair falling across her eyes. She shakes the hair away, but a strand remains moored at her mouth. "'I'd like to take you out,'" she repeats back to him, the hair moving with her lips, curving just beneath her jaw like a brunette moon. "Isn't that what sharpshooters say, *I'm going to take you out*, when they're going to kill you?" She keeps the piece of green foam atop the surface of the water in the bucket. It burbles a moment and then is quiet. He becomes quiet, too, appraising her. He looks at the foam darkening with water. He doesn't want to play with her—they're not teenagers —he doesn't have five minutes more before he has to be on the freeway. "I don't date," she says finally. "I'm sorry." She pulls the oasis dripping from the bucket and lets the excess water drain before she walks back into her table and centers the oasis on the salver. "I'm flattered that you've noticed my flowers," she says. "Thank you," and the intonation is such that he knows he's been dismissed, though dismissed politely.

The handle of the elevator grille feels very cold as he pulls it open to get on the lift. He wonders how many hours she spends up here every day, alone. He had first seen the christening, the tiny roses sewen on the baby May's clothing, the chapel draped with vines. Then he'd seen the book of her work at Rizzoli, had bought it for his mother, for himself, page after page of work without vases, without containers, the flowers and greenery emerging as though growing from the corners of fireplaces, creeping along windowsills, rootless, originless—the Summer Arrangements. His mother had turned the pages with amazement, sometimes greatly amused, commenting finally that this one was so odd, so strange, so good, something evocative of childhood, of hiding in places where one could either overhear or view the goings-on of adults, "striking," she said, "uncanny," the arrangement vining out of the ornate grillwork of the heating register, ivy, woodbine, jasmine trails, red peony and astilbe and blue scabious. He thinks of that arrangement now as he looks through the grille of the lift, thinks he might somehow be that curious, vigilant child within a wall, peering out through a heating register, through vines and flowers, at a woman just beyond. She pulls her foot away from the bucket of sweet peas and props it on the rung of her stool. Then she does something that surprises him greatly: She looks up and waves at him briefly with one small, nervous hand, one small fidgety bird.

As he sinks in the lift, he sees a page from her book. It's a bodice of forget-me-nots, of the tiny blue flowers intricately sewn onto a white silk dress. The flowers garland up and around the young woman's face shadowed by the coffin lid, a very small, narrow garland, as though it is the edge of a mantle, a woodland mantle just starting to cover her.

He cannot decide whether he admires Alice Samara's sense that beauty be remembered as kin to death, or whether he finds this funeral arrangement wholly vain, and then ghoulish and macabre. He doesn't know what he thinks or feels. He supposes he admires her for imagining such an arrangement, for having the nerve to execute it, and then, most bravely of all, for including it in her book. On the opposing page, she had placed a small daguerreotype of a mother holding her dead child, and in the infant's tiny hands rests a nosegay of sweet william. The mother's face appears solemn, but her sadness—certainly evident in the picture—seems somehow lightened, too, by this moment of recording, this presentation of a child she has brought into the world, an event that she insists very quietly on being part of the register. He admires Alice Samara's convictions; he finds them pedantic at the same time.

Forget-me-nots, love-lies-bleeding, Solomon's seal, *Alchemilla*—he has learned from her book the names of the flowers she uses in her arrangements, and some of the lore surrounding them, but as the elevator jolts to a stop, he looks through the sliding grille at a bucket of flowers whose name he does not know, tall-stemmed, richly purple flowers. "What are these called?" he asks Janey as he steps off the lift, and the note of displeasure in his voice cannot be held back.

"Monkshood," she says evenly. Her black-blond hair spikes about her head like gilded thistle. "Blue *Aconitum*," she adds, looking closely at him. She holds yellow pencils in both hands, and a column of numbers mounts beneath each lead. She seems to be calculating supplies needed for some event. Suddenly, like lightning, jagged, flashing, he hates that she can continue to tot up numbers while looking at him, and then, just as rapidly, his anger softens and he feels merely frustrated, and closed in, the flower buckets too numerous and defining too narrowly where he can walk. Foxglove brushes his pant leg and branches of something very tall and yellow-petaled come to his waist. I could give a fuck what *you're* called, he thinks. He nods at Janey, feeling the muscles pull in his neck. "Thank you for letting me go up," he says, "but obviously I didn't pass the test."

Janey lays her pencils down and stands up off the tall stool. "I didn't know you'd gone up there *to* pass a test," she says, and then she puts the palm of her hand against her forehead. "Shit, you didn't, did you?"

"Didn't what?" he asks.

"You didn't ask to see her again, did you? Something like that? You told me you just wanted to tell her how much of a fan you were, something psychiatric about her work. Why'd you do that just now? I thought you wouldn't do that—that you'd give things a little time."

"I have to go," he says, "but I'd like some flowers for Albertine, something she'll like. I needed to be on the freeway ten minutes ago—sweet peas, those are pretty."

Janey moves from around the desk and looks down at some buckets. The back of her neck seems particularly red, burned even. "I guess you know where all the sweet pea are," she says, pulling up into the air several stalks of a pale pink flower. Water drips onto her black patent brogans. The droplets look like blisters—he wants them to be blisters. "I guess I do," he snaps. "What are those?"

"Lisianthus. She's a good person, Luke."

He doesn't say anything, hasn't a word in him edgewise just now that serves as polite public expression. *Why'd the guy name his prick Richard? It was long for dick.* Janey holds the bouquet of flowers up and appraises them. She twists her torso about surveying the floor, eyeing one bucket and then another, and then her eye shoots back to the flowers still held aloft in her hand. The lisianthus bow gently on their stems and he thinks the pink petals beautiful against the deep gray walls of the warehouse— sees Alice upstairs, pretty, as she lifts her small hand to wave at him, shyly, her entire body embowered, ficus and sweet pea, ivy, woodbine, the long oaken boards of the loft floor beneath her, leading to her, away from her, holding her aloft as Janey holds lisianthus before him, adding what he thinks is larkspur, or is it delphinium? Purple blues, violet blues— "Something hot pink," he finally manages to say, "maybe some roses."

"You have a good eye," Janey says, looking up at him; "you always did." And he remembers in seeing Janey just now how crazily different her eyes are, one hazeled with all the colors of autumn, and the other steely cool graphite, as though he is looking into the bore of a pistol.

"What did you do to your neck?" he asks. "Looks like someone tortured it."

"Bleach," she states succinctly. "I fucking did it to myself, can you believe that? It's one thing when you can blame someone else; it's another when you should sue yourself. You want these in a vase—didn't I get you vases for the office?"

"Does Mother recognize you when you do stuff like that to your hair? I mean, she must just shriek upon seeing you sometimes." He gestures for her to wrap the flowers in paper.

"She loves it," Janey counters. "She's not the conservative naïf you think she is."

He knows Janey's right about his mother, that his mother is fearless in the face of the contemporary. She and Janey have been friends—are friends—he has to admit it, no condescension or allowances, but actual friends. More than once he'd returned home and found the windows burst open and noise blasting—he hesitates to call it music—from the casements, Janey's noise, and both she and his mother on their knees, leaning over the flower beds, plunging their bulb dibbles over and over again into the soil, baskets of corms and rhizomes and bulbs sitting behind them, waiting to be interred. They have all had a lot of years together, good conscious years, and Luke is grateful for this.

"She misses the way the house looked when you were there more," he says. "Obviously, the flowers don't look the same, but she knew you'd have to strike out sometime." Luke isn't exactly telling the truth right now, but he also never wants Janey to know why Louise really pushed her to be away more, to get a job. "You couldn't be there forever," he adds.

"I could have just worked at the house." Janey smiles. "I

love Geez Louise, that house, but she wanted me to make a life for myself, sat me down, said, 'Look, honey, I can't set you up with a pension, can't provide for you like you could for yourself if you just got the nerve.' You don't know that, do you? You think your mother's sitting around the house pining for some twenty-something companion she had for eight years." Janey hands him the bundle of flowers, the brown paper crackling as he takes them. "How could you go up there and make a pass at her?"

"I take it we're now talking about Alice. I didn't make a pass at her. I asked her out to dinner. Those are definitely different moves, please admit that."

"What did she say?" Janey asks, serious, genuinely curious.

"She said you were to come up and get the boa for Miss Peaseblossom."

"And besides that, Luke?"

"She never goes out? With anyone?" he asks. "No one?" And then for an instant he is struck himself by how drastic dating actually is, and maybe *drastic* is not exactly the right word, because it is often shallow, tittery, too strained to be satisfying, conversations started but hardly taken to the mat for fear of insult, rejection, the other's sense that you might be a moron, such a febrile and plastic exchange of words, use of time. "So, who owns this business, someone else or Miss Samara upstairs sitting there all alone?"

"Luke," Janey says quietly. "Luke. Leave it alone. It's so beneath you not to make sense, or to be petty and angry. Really, it's not you."

Anger makes you stupid, Luke thinks to himself, pushing the rpms, wanting noise, speed, opening the car up into fifth gear. Janey is right—or she is not, he breathes. *Anger can also make you very, very smart.* He will be the latter, as concentrated as a laser. Sometimes he's alarmed at his own hostility, but then as though miraculously there *is* some order officiated from above, some god, a bumper sticker draws his eye and he reads, IF YOU'RE NOT OUTRAGED, YOU'RE NOT PAYING ATTENTION.

Brilliant. All your degrees and you take solace from sentiments pasted across the rear hulk of a sports utility vehicle. He
glances at the dashboard clock, another feature this car has that
not only works but mollifies him. He's not late; in fact, he's in
the curious and unfamiliar position of having a few abstracted
moments in the middle of the day. He presses the automatic
dial and listens to Albertine answer his office telephone. He
likes the gravity in her voice, always has. He could not stand
someone with a chirp. No one wants to hear game show when
they are calling for an appointment with him, the doctor most
parents call as a last resort, really, actually, a kind of resignation:
I got a kid with a fucked-up brain. He is the doctor approached
when parents have finally admitted *it isn't a phase*, nor is it some
manifestation of their child having turned two years old. And
it's not because this miniature mechanistic monster is a boy
and, you know, boys will be boys. It's not even ADD, this
decade's trendy acronym; no, in fact this kid's got an attention
span like a percussion player in a symphony orchestra. Thank
God for Albertine, who knows just how to receive those initial
calls, just enough facility to put them at ease, to make it seem as
though their office represents possibility, hope, but never so
much that there is a suggestion of a simple cure.

"It's Luke. Do you have your lunch with you today?" he
asks.

"I hate that speaker phone—you sound like you're at the
bottom of a toilet. *Are* you at the bottom of a toilet?"

"Albertine, I'm driving."

"Driving back here, I hope. You've got a full docket. Where
are you stopping for our lunch?" she then asks, because she
knows better than anyone that he is driving back to the office.

Albertine's a big woman and Luke likes the fact that she
likes to eat. He likes to eat, too, and so many times after an
evening out with a woman who has micromanaged some poor
chef's food, Luke has thoroughly enjoyed Albertine's apprecia-
tive ease with food, with *eating* food, with making food. Last
week in the office, he told her about a date he'd had the evening
before. "She orders a stuffed loin of pork without the stuffing

and without the sauce." Albertine just shook her head sadly as she pulled the door closed after her, and then beyond the glass, Luke heard her burst into deep-throated laughter. Luke has never been sure just exactly how many people or issues that particular mirth incorporated as its target.

"Anything sound particularly good?" he asks her now, hoping she will tell him if it does.

"Where are you?"

"On the Ten at Washington."

"Too far for Uncle Darrow's," she laments. "Not much good when it's cold anyway."

"You don't even eat Uncle Darrow's—" he says, but before he can bust her on fried catfish and po'boys, food she did not grow up on, she cuts him off.

"Sushi?" she ventures, and Luke is happy she has. Albertine loves sushi, but he does not think she treats herself to it much because of its expense.

"You have time to call Ariake?" he asks. "I'll come up Olympic."

"*You* have time to call," she says to him gently, almost sweetly, "but I'll do it."

The habit of importance, he thinks, and he has it bad, and the habit of having no time, that habit, too. What can he say? So he does not say anything, shrugging off Albertine's teasing with the anticipation of coming through the door—flowers under one arm, lunch under the other. His colleagues don't care for Albertine, and Luke knows this, and it amuses him immensely. She disturbs the deference ceded doctors, that too-ready subservience people fall into, almost a hush, which Luke hates and which Albertine toys with and complicates constantly.

"You got a nasty bit of horror before Polly," she says, "and Dr. Stieler's office has yet to send over the MRIs. I've talked to the mother four times this morning already."

"It's okay," Luke says. "I'm not sure why they're insisting on seeing me before I have all the files anyway—you think Ariake is open yet?" he asks abruptly.

"For you, Doctor, anytime—you just say when!"

"Yeah, yeah, see you soon."

He can't remember the last time he picked up lunch for Albertine —or for himself, for that matter—and took it into the office. He has flowers brought in all the time—he is his mother's son—and they're right, he thinks, right about the dimension flowers bring to a space, the movement—*they*, he chides himself—*they*, the other species, huh, Luke? *They*, the girls?

He sits at the sushi bar, facing toward the dining room, its tables. The traffic of Olympic Boulevard surges past just outside the immaculate windows. He watches the waiter fill soy sauce pots and remembers reading that the Japanese people originally comprised several different tribes. The waiter is dark-skinned, with a gather of thick black hair down his back. It's tied with a leather thong and a carved piece of wood, ebony perhaps. The tail of the waiter's hair looks—against his white shirt—like a brush stroke of calligraphy. Luke wonders if he would know the man was Japanese if he were lifted from the context of this restaurant. Perhaps he would, because the man looks like a darker-skinned Toshiro Mifune in *Throne of Blood* or *Rashomon*. Yes, Luke affirms, I'd think he was Japanese, but he looks so different from the chef behind the bar, who is tall and round-faced and flat-nosed and pale-skinned. Would Luke know *he* was Japanese?

Lifted from context. It's something Luke has been thinking a lot about, or at least about *context*, how it's created, or not, as in the incapacity of many autistics to create context, a central coherence. He's been poring over Uta Frith again on relevance theory, her contention that autistic children have an inability to process information in context for meaning, and that if they can, the context they create is a bizarre one. Luke supposes an autistic could not manage to be a film editor, could not find and then extract a story from fifty hours of footage. Of course, fiction does not tend to appeal to autistics anyway, and so they rarely understand the conventions of storytelling. What would a film edited by an autistic look like? How fascinating that could be, he thinks, and then he wonders if he'd done the wrong thing by driving downtown, if he'd taken himself so far from context that he seemed absurd, illegitimate, a doctor, mid-morning, walking through the door with nothing better to do than suggest there's a connection between Hiroshima and flower design: Hey, wanna hang, Alice? We can talk bombs and bulbs!

Does she eat sushi? Sashimi? Would she ever sit across a table and eat it with him? Not likely. Though just a few hours ago, driving east on the 10, he'd entertained hopes, even about this evening. Too many hopes, it would now seem.

He'd lost the energy for romantic pursuit a long time ago. A certain set of perceptions has made his desire unseemly to himself, not so much the desire for her, for Alice Samara, but for a companion. He's a doctor, he has money, he drives a beautiful car—all this makes him eligible socially in what are for him the most repugnant of ways. Or maybe not repugnant, but immature. A twenty-two-year-old might flaunt these trappings, might welcome this slick iconography that projects God knows what about him, Luke, the human being, but for Luke it removes him from the equation. And Luke's not very interested in whoever minds cars and titles might factor importantly. He doesn't want to be the emanation of a profession, an automobile company, a financially constituted class. He's not *that* lonely, and yet he's a hypocrite of the highest order, too, as he could not be more willing to have Janey hawk his wares to Alice Samara—anything to get beyond what society thinks his bachelorhood at thirty-seven suggests: an emotional disability, perhaps one bordering on perversion, illness, sexual confusion, of which—as he stiffens thinking about her—he knows he has none.

Sometimes though, sometimes he wishes he had just a little something that complicated his conventionality—not just the fact that he is still unmarried—but something that his blunt uninflected heterosexuality could, in fact, get pointed up with, a little fancy tile work, drapery, some flourish that made him interesting. He would take the consequences, of which there were plenty: legions of men who had nothing to say to you, the "so let me get this straight" look, "There's *no* sport that you follow?" and the complete terror of incomprehension in their faces as Luke lifted his arms into a flamenco position and stomped his feet! Okay, maybe he wouldn't take up flamenco dancing—that might even ride up his crotch a bit—but something to rattle the bars of the ridiculously cramped cage of male heterosexuality. Most women, he regrets, most women when looking for lovers, were as afraid of seeing that cage rattled as are heterosexual men.

But that's not the problem, either, and he knows it, and he feels sad sitting here, aware very clearly of the problem—his problem—and his unwillingness, or fear, maybe that is what it is, fear, to actually divulge in detail, emotional detail, his past to someone with whom he might imagine a future. He keeps himself a cipher, because if someone actually knew how deep and abiding his sadness, would she ever hook her wagon to his? And why? Why take on that load? A lover with a dead sister, and a profession chosen because of it, and a mother whom he protects from the past as much as he can. Alice Samara knew nothing about him, but enough to say no, even to a date. But maybe, he thinks, maybe it's a policy for her and not a response to him? He actually trusted Janey to tell her good things, maybe even interesting things, but then again maybe Janey hadn't said a word. He doesn't really know.

The sushi chef speaks a rapid series of words that Luke cannot decipher and he asks for the chef to repeat them, but the chef lifts a round plastic tray up for Luke to see and it's a composition of bright and subdued color, smelt roe orange and maroon maguro, the different whites of rice and giant clam and halibut, and shapes round and oblong, organic and then the quite purposefully formed. "Yes," Luke says, "yes, beautiful. Maybe a couple of hand rolls?" And the chef lifts a smaller tray of three dark rolls, each with long tails of lurid orange gobo root. They nod at each other, the language of food good and clear and uncomplicated, or at least now in this moment, uncomplicated.

Albertine is printing out the notes Luke took during a session some time ago with a five-year-old boy and his mother, notes that interrupt themselves halfway through with the comment: "We are having an earthquake of some magnitude, maybe a 5.6 or 5.7. Subject: Martin Deliberte, nonresponsive, masturbating, fails to differentiate quake from own body's sensations. Encapsulated. Segmented."

Distracted, Luke lays the bouquet of flowers across the top of the computer. He's reading his notes, the history he took of the pregnancy and of the parents' breakup during Martin's third year of life. He has the school psychologist's recent evaluation, two sets of Griffiths tests and ITPA scores, and an earlier lengthy letter from the father's parents stating their reasons for never wanting to baby-sit Martin again. He'd like to meet these grandparents, as the observations are strikingly detailed, their recording of their grandson's drawings, his language, his malicious behavior, and then, unfortunately, their suggestion of sexual impropriety on the part of the mother, the source—they claim—of Martin's continuous genital fondling. Where else could a three-year-old have learned it but from her? they ask. If it were only as easy as learned behavior, Luke thinks. He realizes the painstaking detail of the letter is so that it might be used in divorce proceedings. He supposes a lawyer's advice is behind it.

"That computer heat sure is good for these flowers," Albertine says. "Nonetheless, I suppose you'll want to put them in some water?" But then Albertine looks up and can see that he is not teasable just now. "Are you going to take him on?" she asks, rising from her chair. She holds the flowers out before her as she walks to the galley kitchen. "These are fine, Lucas, just fine. I love this pink lisianthus."

"How do you know what that's called?" he asks.

"You think your mama has all the books. We called it prairie gentian when I was growing up, but I have come to learn in this great land called Los Angeles: *lisianthus*. You must talk like the folk."

"What do you think?" he asks.

"Two Leiter IQs, one eighty-five a year ago, and ninety-five two months ago—that's not hugely promising," she says.

"Yeah—"

"Wonder what the WISC will show," she adds quickly. "That could profile him well above average, yes?"

These are the more difficult decisions Luke must make.

There are no guarantees, but the higher the IQ, the higher the possibility of success, but sometimes, he hates admitting, the more spectacular the failure, too. Martin would entail three sessions a week for a duration of three to four years, probably much longer. That's a lot of money. "Insurance, the mother's parents," Albertine says without being asked. Who foots the bill, how it all gets paid for, is Albertine's domain.

Luke sits with parents, often grandparents, too, and he gives them this dire prognosis. Even with children for whom he is hopeful, he remains guarded in speaking with the family. He prepares them for the very real possibility of protracted treatment without result. He wonders if it's distinctly American, this desperate equation of money and progress. Oddly, amazingly, the family usually says the right things in response: "We don't expect miracles," or, "If our child's overwhelming anxiety is relieved, it will be worth it—if the panic and tantrums are gone—well then anything, Doctor, anything." But "anything" is not what they mean, and Luke knows this, or maybe anything but the thousands of dollars they will have to cobble together each year from somewhere. It's an exhausting, inscrutable, and very expensive hand they have been dealt, and Luke understands that the money, what it is going to cost, is the one assured thing they have to grasp on to, to particulate clearly, adamantly, and that because it is quite succinctly what they can do, and how they can do it, the money is presented with an unavoidable expectation. It's as though they can't help themselves. All the hope a family has generated and regenerated and insisted upon rides on those dollars, those *few* dollars, Luke wants to emphasize, the price of a car, but knows he must not. Luke doesn't oversee financial matters with the families; Albertine sees to all of this. And this is a good thing, as Luke would have a hard time establishing without seeming defensive that treatment and its progress—or lack of—are distinct, discretely so, from the ever-mounting cost of treatment. One thing is assured: *This will be expensive, and probably forever*; the other thing, treatment, is the best that he—a professional in the field—can do in treating this particular child's psychopathology, listening as carefully as he can for the amount of time he is allowed.

Albertine, standing where a patient or parent might come to stand after entering the office, twists the vase this way and that way on her desk. Some aspect of the arrangement displeases her. Because Albertine is facing her desk, not sitting down behind it, Luke can see a copy of a Bible underneath her chair. It's what Luke believes is called a "presentation Bible," bound in white leather, with a zipper and a small brass cross hanging from its pull. He doesn't know why the Bible is here, and, even more particularly, why is it on the floor. He worries that it might be embarrassing if he were to ask about it.

"I think the sushi chef made us a pretty good lunch," he says, but his words fall flat, seem insincere, forced. A Bible? he wonders. On the floor? Are Bibles supposed to be placed on floors? Albertine will put their lunch on plates and carry the plates into his office where there are chairs, a couch, a small table. He's not eaten lunch with her in a long time and he is looking forward to it. He eats alone often enough that when he shares a meal with someone, it's noteworthy. It's more than just company, though; it is Albertine's company, ironical, funny, intuitively reliable about all manner of things he needs reliable counsel on. He'll ask Albertine about her son in the Coast Guard, any new amazing adventure he might have had recently along the San Juan Islands. Luke will ask Albertine about patients, their parents, about what she hears in the waiting room, what she observes. He supposes he will not ask her about this Bible. As he glances at it again, he notices that her chair's casters are pushed up against it. He still holds the notes on Martin Deliberte as he enters his office. He leaves his office door open. The telephone is ringing behind him and he wants Albertine to allow the service to pick the call up, but she does not and he hears her strong, serious voice. The call is about Martin and she is telling the person on the other end that the doctor "needs to spend some time with the file: he'll call inside a week." "They are anxious, anxious, anxious," she calls from the kitchen, and when she sets their plates on the child's table in his office, she says, "I wanted to look up that place in the Bible where supposedly the word *onanism* springs from—I've never seen a kid masturbate like that Martin. You better help the little guy out."

There is a pun in that, Luke thinks, but he listens only to what he knows she means. He's not much in the mood for humor, or puns or gaiety, but he is in the mood to sit with Albertine for a time. Warm, solid, ingenuous Albertine. *Talk like the folk* Albertine. He has simply loved her for a long time, that little bit of distance she pulls him to, *prairie gentian*, what a beautiful name, and then the compassion she so often reminds him to have in the face of his harsher and more than likely more realistic predictions about patients. But realism is what he and parents have got a surfeit of. Albertine has a type of faith that comes only through the imagination, or maybe it's the heart—Luke does not think he knows—but it sets aside the world and the fire the world is always holding people's feet to. "Oh yeah, that big old fire, it sure is there, but somedays you just turn your scrawny back on it," and Albertine lands a hand heavily on his shoulder and twists him about, turns him away from the fire to face what might be there to be guarded, saved. She doesn't really talk like that—she has a more ironical delivery—but it is what she does for him, for others, to remind them solidly, sensibly, that perspective matters, that hope matters, particularly in light of the situation.

"I always have a time getting used to the patients with those thin, high voices," she says. "Emmett had a voice like that, remember?" And Luke sees that she is reminding him of a patient who now attends Brown, a prestigious university, a patient Luke has helped. The maguro melts across his tongue, flesh that has lived in deep, deep water. Emmett, how is he doing onshore? Luke wonders. How is he getting along?

"Polly, do you want me to sit down?" Luke asks, a little sick at heart that he still doesn't know the right course of action with respect to this tiny chair pushed out from Polly's table. He senses that for Polly, language sheds far too much attention on her thoughts and actions, engenders a painful self-consciousness that places her at a remove, on view. It seems to Luke that for Polly to transform her desires into language gives them a publicity that calls into question her ability to act on them. These ideas, he is well aware, are contrary to thinking about echopraxia. Polly does not wish to appoint herself via language; he's sure of it, sure that this form of objectification doesn't characterize life to her—not her life at least. When she repeats words, it's to push them away, to deflect them, to return them to those who think them operative. She will not claim herself with language; he's sure of it.

The pink daisy on the chair at Polly's table floats far below Luke's eyes. He will be eating his knees, but he takes a chance. He squeezes himself sideways through the closet door, lowers himself onto the tiny chair seat, and leaves his legs stretched beyond the jamb. He attends in the corner of his eye to Polly's small square hands moving slowly over the beads in a blue footed box with a hinged lid. She strokes their glazed surfaces as though comforting them, settling them into some kind of necessary quiet he understands that she projects. The beads, and there are thousands here, are parts of her own body. He is fairly sure that her work at this table is an attempt to make the various parts of her cohere, and that her weaving beads together on her loom is an even more obsessional campaign. She fears fragmentation. She ignores Luke completely. They are alone together.

Then she closes the lid of the blue box and he sees the butterfly raised from its surface. She rubs her fingers frantically across its wings. She then busies herself moving boxes and vials, arranging the table. After every repositioning, she rubs the butterfly again. Luke has never seen her do this before and surmises the butterfly is some kind of safety, a response to his presence so close. He has warned the Markenses that Polly may still spin out at home at any time in response to her table not being there. It does not matter that the table has been here for sometime now. He's unsure, but hopes that Polly's fear of physical obliteration may be soothed by safeguarding what is to her the coherent fixity of this table. Whether she will continue to perceive his office as capable of that safeguarding is another question? And then, of course, it is not here, at the office, where she most needs to be assured of her entirety.

The lowering sun edges a dense, contemplative light in across his office carpet. He sits at the desk with his back to the window—*Backlit*, he thinks to himself—starting the semantical sums and divisions, the linguistic taking apart that he's done ever since graduate school. Years ago, reading for the first time the case of a young autistic girl, and in a similar afternoon light, he'd thought details of the profile made up, fabricated fancifully by a narcissistic doctor for reasons of professional display. But now, after more than a decade of listening, he doesn't think so, doesn't think the case history sufficiently dull to have come from a doctor's mind: A patient, intent upon absolutely every detail of the weather, obsessional for years, divulged to her doctors, much later and almost recovered, that she had lived in terror of being devoured, that *weather*, the word, taken apart, spelled—moreover, profoundly *meant to her*—we/eat/her.

Luke writes *florist* on a tablet of paper. Then in the strong, brisk strokes with which he sets out his letters, he writes flo/wrist; he writes *Alice*, then writes all/ice. He writes *designer*, then writes design/her; he writes *floral*, then writes . . . what? Oral? Floral? Floor/all, flow/all.

He watches Polly in the two mirrors they have now mounted to reflect as well as possible her activity within the closet. They've changed her appointment times so there's no problem with sunlight hitting the mirrors, no sudden silver absence in the glass, and he sees Polly's hands move concertedly, stroking the beads, and though he can't be sure from this vantage, it appears she's setting them all in one direction, marshaling them to rest in lines within their containers. It still amazes him the extent to which an autistic child will go to cement a wall against common experience, against anything that requires confirmation by others. "They're so powerful," he murmurs almost silently, because he is shamed also by his sentimentality. Yet it has to be noted, this will to omnipotence these children have. Childhood is perhaps a terrible condition for such powerful persons to be locked within . . . add the confinement of public school to that, and Luke fears for all involved.

He fingers in from memory the telephone number for Delmonico's on Pico. Earlier, he'd had the absurd fantasy of dining there tonight with Alice Samara, a booth with the curtains pulled, as private a dinner experience as one could have in this town of gated homes but fishbowl restaurants. "Yes," he says when the hostess comes on the line, and then he says, "Sure," but he is saying it to no one, because she has pushed the hold button even before her own words are completely spoken: "Would you please ho—"

It's part of the gestalt of L.A. The willingness to be treated like shit as long as one is treated in this manner by someone who might give one what one wants. Is there a pervasive erosion of social etiquette? His patients have a difficult time perceiving social conventions, certain niceties. Perhaps this is becoming a more general problem?

When the hostess comes back on the line, it's hard for Luke because he knows her, likes her, can see her angularly thin body in its fashionable garments, the rock-star cross hanging in the niche of her throat. Keep your eye on the prize, he thinks. He just wants a booth at the back of the restaurant, and anyway, Lordy, where would he start in an attempt to explain why this phone style is not—and then that's just it: It is not even style; it's bad behavior gotten up as style and rationalized by the insisted-upon necessity of speed. Luke, *Luke*, just get yourself a table for dinner, man. A whiz and a bang, eye on the prize, just get your business done.

She greets him with Delmonico's large menus clasped against her chest, her chin resting on the menus' top edges, a practiced illumination in her eyes. She speaks briskly, brightly, that gaiety of kindergarten teachers, which is usually not warmth. Though he comes here once a week at least, he's sure that her recognition is completely visual, that she doesn't retain his name. He

wonders if she does it for a reason, elides any deeper acknowledgment. She's got to be hit on all the time, Luke thinks, by
young and old. He wonders if she ever says to them, "I'm sorry,
but I don't date." He wants to ask her whether she knows anyone who does not date, who just refuses the ritual. How do you
get to audition with someone like that, Cheryl? he wants to ask,
using her name, which he has known for some time now. He
watches her clipped sashay ahead of him as she makes her way
down the aisle between the booths and the tables. He decides
she has a bit of a strange figure, broad, flat hips, which do not
exactly seem to scale with the rest of her very thin body. He
manages to be looking at her face when she stops and swivels
around to indicate the booth she is seating him in. Do not
say it, he coaches her silently. Say something totally different, a
comment about storm-drain construction or Frederick's of
Hollywood going bankrupt, anything but "enjoy your dinner!"
which you could give a flying leap about. Come on, Cheryl, he
urges, liking her manicured nails, drop the automation, say
something off script.

"Will anyone be joining you this evening?" she asks, and
Luke has to snicker at himself, the one question, off script or
on, he would rather not have had tossed up in his face, particularly this evening. Baby, have you ever seen anyone *join* me for
dinner, let alone walk through the door with me?

"I only date women who don't date," he says a bit too
tersely, though he has meant to be jocular, amusing, open to
approach, the nasty soliloquy in his head that of another man
entirely. She thinks he's pathetic and he knows this from the
painful smile her lips press out. He bends down into the booth
and then stretches his legs out across the floor to the other
banquette.

"I guess I don't get it," she says apologetically.

She hands him the wine list and lays the menu across his
bread and butter plate. He expects her to leave, but she does
not. Brunello, he is thinking as he opens the wine list, but he
says, willing the terseness into his voice this time, "Irony? You
don't get irony?"

He looks up, to see the smile drop from her face, and she says, "No, of course I get irony. I don't get why women don't date you."

This is not the conversation he wants to have right now, and definitely not with Cheryl the hostess, though why she deserves his condescension, he's not sure. It's not as though *she* broached the issue of dating, and here she is standing over him, lovely to most eyes, handing him an opening on a platter and—for his serving ease—a meat fork. Excellent, Luke, top of your form, he says to himself. Care to come up with some tact right about now? He hopes to hell someone writes her a mash note soon to make up for what he is about to do.

"Would you mind sending the waiter over," he says casually, a casualness that suggests with a mallet, I didn't hear what you just said and I most certainly reject its kindness. And then, because he is hating himself, he adds, in the voice of a doctor he could package and sell, "Thank you, Cheryl; it's always nice to see you."

The restaurant is virtually empty. It is early. Luke rhymes *hating myself* with *dating myself,* but he doesn't hate himself; he just doesn't like to hurt people's feelings. Hard to argue, however, that I'm not dating myself, he thinks.

"How are you tonight, Doctor?" The waiter stands looking down at the page of the wine list Luke is reading. Luke knows him, a comfortable, affable boy on his way to med school, but enjoying the scenery while he's at it.

"What the hell are we drinking tonight, Mark?" Luke says by way of hello, exhausted, but also instantly, unconsciously at ease talking to a man.

"Something red?" Mark asks. "That Antinori Chianti's nice."

"How's a Brunello sound?"

"You got it," the waiter says. "See the news?" he asks, opening Luke's menu for him. "Medics had to cut a boa constrictor off a pregnant woman today—seems she was trying to get over her fear of snakes by sleeping with one."

"We do prevail, we do prevail," Luke says, laughing, and then Mark gets it, too, and laughs.

"Yeah, man, but they had to cut it off her."

What's so new about that? Luke thinks, and Alice Samara is in his sights again, her foot propped up on the stool rung, the small black shoe—he wants to make it elfin, but it's not; it's just a small black shoe with a low heel that curves in elegantly—and he's so far gone on that shoe, the woman wearing it, the arms suspended above the table, working deftly, a white sweet pea blossom fused with a pink, then with another white, another pink, the garland becoming beneath her fingers as active as hands jerking him off, and he thinks he would have to calm her, says, Jesus, baby, not so fast, you're not whipping egg whites, then the fingers slowing, holding him tightly, the small small fists wrapped around him working themselves into quiet, efflorescence.

Stan has been shouting, roving about the office as Luke sits on the carpet by the drafting table, but now Stan decides he will draw, and so he assiduously positions the green pencil in his fingers, both his hands held up so as to block Luke's vision of his face. When he lowers his hands and starts to move them above the paper, his eyes gaze well past Luke, seemingly past—or through—any obstruction this building's walls might present. An idea suddenly occurs to Luke, occurs to him perhaps because he's been thinking about Alice Samara's work—because he's thought more about her rejection of traditional floral structures, vases and pots and corsages. There's the appearance in so much of her work of the flowers being airborne, fluid, apparitional, the appearance that the arrangement is not moored anywhere specific or stable. Stan's drawing is three-dimensional, is not moored upon or by paper—not even, for God's sake, by lines. What if Luke were to put Stan in a dark room with a laser, one of those pointers used in presentations with overhead projectors? He wonders how Stan would react to an actual visual manifestation of what his hand makes when it moves, whether it might allow him a stronger sense of the drawing and writing, of making something in the world. Of course, the laser's beam would last only for a few seconds before disappearing, but it'd be there for a time nonetheless.

"How do you feel about being in the dark, buddy?" Luke asks Stan, though his question fades because he sees that Stan is clutching his crotch with one hand as the other continues to sketch above the page. Luke unfolds himself from the floor and then reaches across his desk into the kneewell. He buzzes Albertine so that she can take Stan to the bathroom, but there is no answer. It's not a good thing for him to attend to Stan, to blur the distinction between parent and doctor, but Luke also wonders if maintaining this distinction now, in this instance, might be totally bogus, too. Were Luke to stand and urinate beside Stan—both of them happily doing so— it might secure an identity between them, each enough like the other to engage in common behavior—in other words, *in play*, an activity that exactly depends upon this commonness. Pee therapy, Luke thinks seriously, dismally, but he remembers vaguely an old old case, maybe forty years old now, that documents a little girl who came to understand play by urinating in her counselor's lap one day. The counselor did not get angry, had, in fact, been carefully trained not to show displeasure with respect to issues of elimination, and so she actually smiled, and because of this, the girl seemed to think the counselor and she had wet themselves at the same time, that they had done this together, enjoyed it together. Luke understands that the counselor smiling at that precise moment had miraculously made the difference, had secured at last a common goal for both patient and therapy. The little girl improved from that point on, the counselor's smile a lucky, lucky response. Luke doubts he would smile were Stan to casually urinate on him, *or* on his floor. He buzzes for Albertine again. Stan's face is stiffening with anxiety.

"Okay, Stan the man—seems we need to use the facilities. Let's go do it."

They pass through the outer office, through the vague scent of roses, and walk down a long hall to the point at which it forms an ell. Stan has been striding eagerly beside Luke, moving swiftly but as Luke makes the turn, Stan bounds straight into the wall. "Rejected. Not tactical to travel forward in a single line," he says sternly, and then doubles over in uproarious laughter.

Luke laughs, too. What is he going to do with this kid? He can see a very young Frank Sinatra saying this in the movie, just before they're betrayed by their scout, but Luke doesn't think Stan's actually alluding to imminent peril so much as he is just having a goof on the wall being there. But a typical kid would have done this with slapstick alone; Stan did it with language.

Luke presses a code into the keypad near the bathroom door and it clicks once. Stan pushes in against the door, opening it a couple of inches, and then stops. He holds his child's hand up as though to stop traffic. "Having been relieved of those uniquely American symptoms, guilt and fear, he cannot possibly give himself away." Stan lets the door close and Luke hears its mechanisms lock. "We're going through this elaborate procedure simply out of precaution in case there are any visitors."

Luke thinks that certainly one very clear reason not to leave his office with a patient is because he is away from his notes and the tape recorder. Stan's lines are coming quickly and Luke is shuffling through the movie's scenes as rapidly as he can, trying to place the lines, who speaks them, the context. Stan looks up at Luke, shows Luke his small hands, front and back, a magician about to dupe an audience. He then keys in the code for the bathroom door and pushes it all the way open this time. Five digits. How Stan knows the digits is not what Luke is thinking about so much as the fact that Stan is making commentary on the absurd secrecy of a bathroom with a coded keypad. Stan runs from urinal to urinal, crouched, an invader across enemy lines. He looks back, his eyes surveilling, waves his arm to Luke to move forward, signaling, the coast is clear; I've got you covered. Just then a toilet flushes loudly and as the stall door swings open, Stan is startled. "I was first in line until the little hairball was born," he shouts, looking up disdainfully at Luke, though Luke knows the disdain is not for him. Stan was having a good time, but now his shoulders are down around his waist and his mood is as suddenly dark as an oven after its interior light has been switched off.

The man who has come from the stall is dressed in a dark blue suit, its fabric drawn taut across his beefy back. He doesn't acknowledge Luke or Stan. He looks at himself in the mirror over the sinks. He doesn't wash his hands, but as they reach to worry the wide rep tie, Luke sees a silver class ring with a blue stone on his right hand. The man is all of a piece, Luke thinks, so much so that he probably has rotten molars from sucking breath mints. He's a salesman and his cases are sitting in some office's reception area. Luke takes note of his class ring again, tries to see the school, but why he doesn't really know; he'll think about that later. Now, he wants the man at least to acknowledge Stan's presence, a nod of the head, a muttered hello.

Stan moves to the low urinal and tugs his pants and underwear down around his knees and begins to urinate. "The buzz from the bees is that the leopards are in a bit of a spot," he intones without inflection. The door to the bathrooms closes and Luke moves to the urinal beside Stan's and gazes distractedly at the stream of urine from his penis, the silly corkscrew to the left that hits the top of the pink deodorizer. "The buzz from the bees is that the leopards are in a spot," Stan says again, no more inflection in his voice than the first time. Luke watches his urine "buzz" into the spots through which it drains. Those connections are probably not at play in Stan's mind, but Luke conjures various conceits nonetheless. Luke's father used to say, "Take the dog out for a whiz and a bang." Luke doesn't remember his family ever owning a dog, but he remembers that sentence, the onomatopoeia, his father saying it. Why he can't remember a dog, the oddness of that, why the man's class ring just caught his eye, Luke's curiosity about it—he will think about this all later. "Do you like that pun, 'the leopards are in a bit of a spot'?" he starts to ask Stan, but Stan is hauling his pants back up and moving to stand before the door. Not only is Stan going to get his face smashed in by an opening door—and so should not wait there—Luke wants him to wash his hands. Whether Stan will move to the sinks willingly or whether he'll have to be moved there by Luke is a guess. Luke examines the difference in Stan's behavior when he's perseverating one movie versus perseverating the other: *The Lion King*—Stan will have to be moved; *The Manchurian Candidate*—he'll move himself.

"Stan, let's wash our hands," Luke says, tucking himself in, smoothing the fly on his boxers. Stan remains steadfast in front of the door. "Stan, if someone tries to come in and that door swings in and hits you, it'll hurt. You'll have a black eye, and then it's anyone's guess who your doctor will be. It'll sound pretty bad when I tell them you walked into a door, or rather, it walked into you. Think they'll believe me?"

Stan is gone into himself, water poured into water, irretrievable, and Luke knows it. He also knows that rarely if ever does rational explanation work with autistic children. Luke moves Stan gently from the door to one of the sinks and then places his hands beneath a faucet. They dangle and move within Luke's hands as though water, too. Luke fears that here in the bathroom amid the hard surfaces, Stan might suddenly toggle into manic activity, hurting himself against the porcelain and tile, but Stan remains underwater—of the water.

In the office again, Stan draws in the sky with his *vert vif* pencil for the rest of the hour. He does not speak other than—upon leaving—to enunciate tonelessly the question, "Why can't he kill some nonproductive person on the outside?"

Luke hears the anxiety of the question in the movie. The doctors are arguing over Raymond Shaw's conditioning, whether his brainwashing is completely reliable. They're going to have Shaw kill somebody as a kind of test, and they're arguing the choice of victims. The frantic doctor who objects to one of his staff being killed speaks from a face oozing sweat and oil.

Luke is pretty sure Stan wouldn't like that face, but does Stan configure himself as Raymond, the brainwashed pawn, ready to be deployed? Or is he, Luke, the witless Raymond about to "kill" Stan, as opposed to some nonproductive person outside his office? Not only does Stan change movies but he changes the characters Luke assumes he's identifying with, or speaking through. Luke's never exactly known what triggers a film change, though he suspects that when Stan feels least powerful, least able, he switches to *Lion King*, to the obvious certainty throughout the film that Simba will grow up and prevail and be king. Today, in the bathroom, when the man had appeared, Stan had used a line of Scar's, the nasty uncle who hates Simba, the heir apparent, but now Stan is back to *The Manchurian Candidate*, and Luke surmises it's because of the curious complication in the film in the character of Raymond Shaw. Un-brainwashed, before his capture by the Communists, Raymond is a son of a bitch, cold, mean, dictatorial. After he's brainwashed, he's not one smidge nicer or kinder or smarter. Only *now*, because of various machinations by the enemy, Shaw is a nationally celebrated war hero. Stan is seven years old, actually eight now—Luke underlines this in his mind—but Stan *gets* irony, and Luke draws an ever-darkening circle around this word in his mind, *irony*. "No autistic kid understands irony," he says aloud to himself, "nope, unheard of"—even Luke is resistent to this refinement in Stan, but he knows there's something about it that's true, too. And he, Luke, is one of the primary sources of irony in Stan's mind. A doctor is not someone to make you well, to make you better, a doctor is a control, someone who wants you to do something you would not do of your own accord. A doctor's face oozes oil and sweat.

Ah, Stan, Luke thinks, as doctors go, I'm a beauty. Come on, admit it, Stan. But in the same plush of Luke musing, of letting his mind drape between appointments, Stan's words rip through like a blade: "Why can't he kill some nonproductive person on the outside?"

I don't know, Stan, I just don't know. Luke enunciates this quietly to himself.

Because it is March, and a tradition, Luke and his mother walk through the greenhouses at Zuma Canyon Orchids. He accompanies his mother every year, and though the excursion is ostensibly to see the phalaenopsis in bloom, the outing also falls during the time of year when Sadie was dying—and then was dead. Neither of them ever make comment about this coincidence—that would be unnecessary, ever indelicate—but of the five orchids his mother traditionally buys, one is for Sadie, will always be for Sadie, his sister. He does not think of her right now in the fetal warmth of the two huge greenhouses, but she is always with him, in him, systolic, a measure in blood of his life.

They walk slowly down an aisle of magenta phalaenopsis, some of the tall flower stalks bowing one way and others bowing another, the richly colored blossoms serried along the stalks and quivering in the gentle commotion of ceiling fans revolving overhead. Louise turns and beckons Luke forward through the long, long aisles of tables covered in plants. "You must choose," she says, and he knows what she means, that this year Sadie's orchid is his choice. "My son has a good eye."

He hears Janey say the same words to him, the feminine version of "You do that just as well as a man," and yet of course it is different because both Janey and his mother take delight in his attention to the beauty that interests them—they're far more egalitarian, no clubbishness but rather this high and welcoming plane. He hears himself, that day he visited Alice Samara's studio, ask rather acidly who owned the business, "Someone else or Miss Samara upstairs," and he hears Janey say, "Luke. Luke. Leave it alone." And he had left it alone, had not called Alice or attempted another trip downtown. He'd driven dutifully down the Santa Monica Freeway that morning, exiting at Robertson, turning up Olympic Boulevard on his way to Century City, the flowers laid across the seat next to him, moist and alive and hopeful. He pulled in at Ariake for sushi. He'd seen Stan Mingis earlier, then later tested a toddler with brain damage incurred when her older brother lost hold of her in a speedboat rising and plopping across a choppy lake. He had spent an hour and a half with the toddler's parents, working hard to persuade them that the older brother needed the most immediate care, but their anger at their son was so consuming, they could only regard him as culpable, a child who had made a mistake and who would have to survive, because to do any less was to somehow usurp his baby sister's identity.

Now, in re-creating this scene, it's the son Luke sees bobbing in the rough water, the son's head sinking, emerging, sinking, struggling weakly, suffering. "My son has a good eye," his mother says to him again, because he's holding a plant out to her, a somewhat small white orchid with a greenish tint, and as his mother gazes intently at its leaves, Luke hears, "*Not* a phalaenopsis, a species, never hybridized, so it still has a detectable odor, *odorat*." The voice speaks the Latin laughing, the same voice that said, "Yes, sweet peas, lots of sweet peas," and he looks up, to see his mother watching Alice Samara across his shoulder, his mother as electrically palpable behind him as Alice Samara is standing miraculously before him, both of them so significantly on either side of him, he feels ecstatic, crazily, stupidly happy, buoyed beyond manners as his mother reaches her hand around him and says, "I'm Luke's mother, and you must be Alice Samara. Please call me Louise." And then, as though he is not there, or is merely smoke, they take and shake each other's hands and then pass before him and walk off together, two small women, one younger, one older, their bodies surrounded by thousands of phalaenopsis plants, white, so many blossoms of velvety white petals shimmering along their stalks, and violet and purple—a daub of yellow blossoms here and there on either side of them.

He takes a moment to calm himself, to extract himself from what now seems a dramatic event pulsing with electrical self-consciousness. It's the beauty of the orchids, the humid comfort of the greenhouse, the serendipity of meeting her again, without effort or design, and his mother, his great mother, reaching a hand out to Alice immediately as though to secure her company. It flashes into his head that that day he'd finally met Alice was a day upon which he'd seen Polly Markens, too, and that it had been a day of progress for him and Polly in that he had felt he'd done something right for her, had understood definitely where the analogue for her body's physical integrity resided, and he had sat down in one of her small chairs and it had been tolerated. Unfortunately, Polly's progress has recently stalled. He thinks it might have to do with Polly having had a sudden growth spurt, her body rogue, out of her control.

"I think Janey misses a more easeful schedule," he hears Alice say to his mother. "We've had too many weddings in Malibu, and I'm a lot less interesting to work for—"

Luke likes hearing Alice Samara's voice, the deep richness from such a small body, and the tone always playing at humor, it seems to him, humor hard-won and necessary.

"Luke bought me your book—" Louise says.

"Oh, that's how you knew who I was—that book! I hate that book. Janey talks about your garden—"

"You must come home with Janey to see it," Louise says now, definitively. "Particularly if you're in Malibu so much."

Luke knows what his mother will do, knows where she's leading, that by the time he drives her back down the gravel and dirt of Bonsall Drive, Alice Samara will be coming to dinner, and he laughs out loud—and loudly—because he can't predict across the distance of the ten feet of tanbark they've walked whether he will be invited or not.

He watches how Alice's breasts move as she turns to see why he laughs. He sees their undulant float beneath the white shirt and wants to remember this movement for a long time. He wants to think of it as gesture, invitation, Alice coming toward him—he's too used to finding great advancement in small actions, progress in a nonresponsive child from the most momentary eye contact. "You're fast friends," he says to Alice by way of explanation. "I was only marveling," and then he says something he has not planned to say, or rather, he will think later, it says itself using his mouth and tongue and palate. "This orchid is for my dead sister." He is still holding the plastic pot and it's small and lightweight and warm against his palm. He can see his mother's face over Alice's shoulder, the perfect complexion of her old skin, her blue eyes as glazed as porcelain—she can't understand why he has said such a difficult thing just now, can't understand why he'd do this to Alice Samara.

"Yes, this is for Sadie," his mother says quickly. "You obviously approve," she adds, reaching with one hand for the green plastic pot and taking Alice's arm with the other, but Alice doesn't turn back or move.

"We buy an orchid for Sadie every year," he says. "You understand that," he adds, and the tone of his voice startles him, and most particularly he is startled by the yearning in his chest, not for Sadie, though that is never absent, but for someone else to know, to share in the ritual of his sister's memory. He understands the tone of his voice is that of someone asking for help. But it is not that, not primarily that; it is connection, something he has divulged that might begin to paint him more fully in her mind. *Divulged*, he thinks. Okay, well maybe he actually lobbed it right at her head, but he does not care to feel chagrined, and all the hearty acceptable male stances in the world will not erase the fact of Sadie's death in his life, in his voice, if that is where she is at the moment.

"It's unusual," she's saying to him, turned slightly, talking across her shoulder, but he doesn't hear what she's saying—or he does—it's audible, audible to him, but her face is careful in her regard of him, and this is what he sees, what he really hears, that she's not scrambling from the emotional difficulty of the moment. She's not glossing past it to some polite social ease. He's managed to interest her by what he's just given her a glimpse of— and *that*, that is in her clear face and in her voice . . . and in the gentle scent of the greenhouse. "Species are my favorites," she is saying, "but you can't really use them that much; they're too small. People don't really see them."

"Don't you think Janey has told your Alice Samara about Sadie?" his mother asks as he drives too fast down Pacific Coast Highway, changing lanes in lieu of changing subjects, license plates coming into perfectly legible view, his mother stiffening just a little each time before he careens his car aside and passes.

"She's not *my* Alice Samara," he says, knowing his mother isn't about to diffuse her focus by discussing his youthful driving. He's shifting in and out of fifth gear for no good reason. The hard wooden knob soothes his palm. Any subject, he's thinking, any subject you'd like, Mother, but this one.

"No, but certainly you're enamored of her," Louise says.

"I embarrassed you, didn't I?" he says. "Back there, in the greenhouse, I embarrassed you by bringing up Sadie." He looks across the car at his mother, her profile against the steel gray of the Pacific Ocean. She is watching the road for both of us, he thinks, but he looks back to the white truck whose tailgate chains rattle furiously over the bumps in the road. The racket of the chains encourages him and he practically drives up into the truckbed before he finally switches lanes. Christ, she's a stoic, he thinks to himself, looking across again, her scarf still perfectly draped, the bracelets, significant, gold, heavy on her narrow wrist as it lies along her knee.

"You seemed a little desperate," she says quietly, and the honesty of what she's suggested dilates in the car as though it were an overhead light switched on, glaring. She's right, of course, and he's heard it himself in his voice, his words. "What was her response when you asked her out," she asks, "when you went to the loft?"

"If you know that much, you know the rest—Janey and you have obviously had a powwow." He slows the car for the light at Temescal Canyon. He's never really minded his mother and Janey talking about him, and yet he's pretty sure their conversations have never been about women, *his* women, though why not, he can't say. A passing comment certainly, even a scathing comment here and there—his mother not particularly given to keeping her perceptions polite—but detailed discussions about his sexual life with women, no. So he's a little surprised, but it's also hardly a full-blown disquisition for Janey and his mother to have exchanged the two sentences it would have taken to divulge that he had indeed asked Alice Samara for her time, and that she had said no.

He doesn't want to be elusive with his mother, doesn't want to be angry with her, nor does he want this viscous shame snailing across his body. "Most men discuss their dating with someone other than their mother," he says, larding some ease into his words, exactly the same winsome, vaguely wooing tone he mastered as a teenager to procure car privileges, charge cards, steaks instead of chicken, airfare.

"That would be their loss," his mother says with certainty in her voice.

He laughs at this, smelling her perfume as he does, a scent so familiar, so abiding, it calms him. "You're probably right."

"She's coming to dinner on Saturday, and with Janey, to see the garden, though, of course"—she pauses, smiling—"though of course you're welcome to cook."

He isn't traveling through the intersection as quickly as the white truck, now behind him, would like, and the horn startles him, and then even more so the look on the man's face in the rearview mirror, a cartoon of rage, livid, bulging cheeks beneath blond buzz-cut hair. Luke wants to apologize to this driver he's menaced, wants to cook for them all. Alice is coming to dinner; he'll never tailgate again. I'm an asshole, he thinks to yell out the window. You're absolutely right, a total asshole, he wants to proclaim gleefully. "Yeah?" he says aloud to his mother, yeah by way of confirmation, *really*? And it's as though he truly is sixteen again, and winsome, and rather a jerk, too, he muses, like most young men that age not yet very clear on the distinction between vigor and aggression.

In the car alongside theirs, a car waiting for the light at the next intersection as Luke and his mother wait, a child in her car seat rivets Luke's eye. She has ahold of her ear in her tiny hand, and she kneads the lobe between her fingers. She regards him seriously, concertedly, almost diagnostically, her little head moving in reception of the comfort of her kneading, her eyes never straying from his. It's called "self-comforting," and he's thought a lot about what he thinks are intensified forms of self-comforting in autistic children. Thumb sucking, ear rubbing, these are milder, less injurious forms of head banging, chest thumping, though making this point is complicated, as one activity is so obviously benign, a complement to parental care, a sweet tick—and the other activity seems a violent rejection of nurture.

Polly's not responsive, and yesterday in therapy he'd had to prevent her from swallowing a Venetian bead she particularly loves. He'd held her during her immense furious tantrum. All the while he'd talked to her of the allure of the beads, their opalescence, their shine—he'd kept racking his brain for words as beautiful and interesting as the beads themselves—incandescent, nacreous, flinty, rubescent, vermiculated, millefiori, celadon. He's always so amazed by the importance of beauty to autistic children, their ecstatic, almost ravenous reception of it, and then often how instantly a tantrum follows. He'd held Polly tightly, her arms and legs pinwheeling . . . and held her somewhat loosely, too, in that he'd wanted to somehow convey to her that her ecstasy wasn't wrong, wasn't something she needed curing of. He wanted her to remain as close as safely possible to her elemental delights, to the sensuality that gave her a sense of physical wholeness. He'd seen the abstracted eggheads intelligent autistic children could become—he questions that "health," defies the accepted idea that completeness can't come from autosensual experience. Obviously it can—so obviously.

"You do what you can do, Luke," his mother says, startling him. He'd been so completely in a place he likes being, thinking about children, thinking them out of their prisons.

"What?" he says, annoyed. "What?" He has no idea why she's said what she's said.

"You desperately want all your children to be healthy, happy—like that child."

"I guess I'm Mr. Desperation today, Christ." The light finally turns green and he depresses the clutch and pushes the stick shift forward into first. It's a sensually engineered car, and it annoys him how much he likes driving it, but he is seduced by it, too, by how sexual he finds it, smoothing it through its paces. How hard it would have been to give up the sleek, powerful body of a horse surging beneath you for those first lurching, chugging, belching automobiles—how impossible. He would have spurned those automobiles, but not this one, not this better part of a century of engineering and design. "She said," he intones, "she said in response to my request—that day I went to see her in her studio—she said she did not date."

"And you took that," Louise asks, "as a definitive no?"

"I have never pushed," he says.

"You mean you have never had to?" his mother says.

"No, Mother, I don't mean— Janey said to leave her alone, to leave it; she said it in such a way that I did. I spend much of my life goading people, children, into doing what they distinctly do not want to do. I don't have much left over for chasing around. I'm sorry if you think me somehow less a man for not breaking down the door and dragging her out by her hair—"

"Yes, and then fucking her into sensibility," his mother interjects, because it will stop him, and because he knows she doesn't even remotely think what he's just accused her of, that he's just on that tired path because it's there, pointed out, an invitation. "Easy, kiddo," she says. "I couldn't respect you more. And incidentally, I love you, too."

He doesn't always know how to respond to his mother, to her rather granite attestations. He knows her feelings, though, has always felt that he knew them, and there's trust within that, and solace.

"Alice Samara waved to me as I was leaving that day. She was working on something—with sweet peas, a garland or something—but she raised her hand, and it was like a little bird fluttering—she has nervous hands—and she unbuttoned and buttoned and unbuttoned her shirt several times, unconscious of it completely, a top button, at her neck—not as I was leaving but during the course of talking. It wasn't sexual; it was nerves."

"You're taking me to dinner somewhere?" Louise asks.

"I am," he says, moving the gearshift forward and then pulling it back, downshifting expertly; he is easy on a car.

"Is she a patient, Luke, or is she someone you want to know in a different way, as a woman?"

He accelerates up the California Incline, and as the car pulls up onto Ocean and becomes level again, no longer laboring, he says quietly, "Now who's being nasty?"

"It's a serious question."

"Of course it's a serious question," he snaps.

"I didn't mean it harshly."

"But you meant it definitively," he says.

The car is quiet, rolling down Ocean Park, and then he tugs the wheel and whips the car neatly around in a U-turn to pull in front of the restaurant and the valets. He pushes the lock button and the mechanism rackets loudly in the doors, which are being opened on both sides as Louise says, "We can't leave these orchids in the car like this. We have to go home first."

He looks down behind the seats into the foot well at the five pots spaced carefully between copses of wadded newspaper. "Are you sure?" he asks, turning forward. The car fills with cold, vibrant sea air. The valets wait, the one on Luke's side looking out across the street, across the civic rose garden, at the ocean, the sun low in the sky. Luke thinks the valet's gaze is less deferential than it is impatient, his face turned aside to hide this. "Mother?" Luke says patiently, his inflection merely a way to establish his mother's wishes.

"It's terrible for them—" she says, moving the clasp of one of her bracelets around her wrist, her tick always, the stagy business of her serious jewelry.

Luke opens the cover over the ashtray and pulls from a small, tight roll a couple of ones. "Guys, thanks, we have to come back," he says easily, handing the bills up to the valet, a soiled, metalic whiff lingering in his nose, the smell of the money intensified by salt air. He has ahold of his door and releases the services of the valet on his side by saying, "Save us a place." He looks across and sees his mother's door being pushed carefully in, an assiduous attention being paid to avoiding fingers or coattails or scarf points. The face of the valet is in the window and Luke can see that he is no older than sixteen, and frightened, an emotion that in time, Luke thinks, will either toggle all the way over to anger or will merely flatten into servility. And somehow Luke knows this isn't an evening job, isn't an after-school, mad-money job for this kid—it's the show. Glancing in the rearview mirror, Luke sees him take a sparring stance on the sidewalk, sending punches into the air at the level of his ears, one two three—boom; one two three—boom. It's a display for the guy in the nice car who can't make up his mind, Luke thinks, a "Fuck you, mister! Don't you dare feel sorry for me." No. It's a round for the valet himself, a throwing off of Luke's glance and of what it took in—what it decided upon. Luke feels sheepish at his own egoism, how far it encroaches, a type of psychological imperialism that comes with the mantle of his profession. He wants to have felt that his empathy means something, *is* something, causes him to be better and to do better things; it doesn't cause much at all—it *means* frighteningly little.

"Not a patient," he says to his mother, looking ahead down the cracked cement of the street, the car moving beneath the crazily lanky palms, "Alice is not that, though how could I not see her flowers a certain way, not think about them?"

"I don't mean that you won't see things," Louise says, "just that your distance from them is not clinical."

"I'm not going to deny that my interest started out that way," he says. "Why should I deny it?"

"Because it's a hell of a sexless way to start a relationship."

He grunts as though he's sixteen. Grunts! The thirty-seven-year-old Luke poof, gone, *desaparecido*. How masterful his mother is at making his older self disappear—or maybe, how powerless he is in the face of his own spontaneous erasure. He isn't the first to be appalled in maturity by just how instantly the child reconstituted, sprang mewling from the older, willful self. Luke supposes he can't claim Louise as having caused it, *done it*, that by this time he had to meet the child he still harbored head-on. But grunting? When had he ever grunted?

As he turns the car up San Vicente, he glances at her. She is smiling again, her wrist held up, her other hand moving the bracelets about. He wonders if Sadie, had she grown up, grown older, would have worn her jewelry like Louise, like her mother, their mother, several bracelets deep, large ones, amusing charms, a few obscene ones bestowed by a European lover to whom Louise was briefly married, and an intricately tooled Greek bracelet in a brighter rendering of gold that had been a gift from Luke's father, a gift scaled, Luke mused, to the possibility that Louise would give up her others. This had not happened. "Quite a totem pole you've got there, Mother," Luke says, feeling at once bold and stupidly young. "May I have one for Alice?"

"When the time comes, yes, of course," his mother says without hesitation, with no whiff of reservation or possessiveness. "But Janey gets the charm bracelet. And don't forget that, you acquisitive little shit."

The blue streaks in his mother's conversation have always been there; he's heard them all of his life, the *shits* and *fucks* and *cocksuckers*, an armature of words surrounding her deeper sentiments. At Louise's cusses, he's seen many a raised eyebrow, a horrified flinch, but he'll take the voluble clarity of his mother's pronouncements, how loud their communications. "You like Alice, don't you? Already protective of her," he says. He feels intrigued that Alice appeals to his mother, even a little relieved, let off some mother-son hook that would seem to guarantee tension. There are the common botanical interests, he thinks, and the solitariness, but really it's something his mother is perceiving in him, something about his reactions to Alice, his silliness in the greenhouse, the tone of his voice telling her about Sadie—that's what his mother has heard, the tone asking for company in a room that has long been airless.

He likes driving down the wooded darkness of San Vicente at night, the huge coral trees overhanging the broad median, and the houses deeply recessed from the street behind old and dense landscaping. It's not dark yet, though, and he laments how much he can see, or perhaps, more so, that he can be seen, that he's not passing swiftly, anonymously down this broad boulevard. Just whom he might be seen by is exactly no one and, simultaneously, of no consequence. He feels this desire to be unseen anyway, some great oxygenated freedom in being an invisible face in a car ducking past, and then gone. But it's still light and his mother sits in the car just inches from him. Never is he less invisible—never is there more of Luke to be seen—than in the presence of his mother. He turns the car off San Vicente and up her street.

"Did you ever know—" he begins to ask, "—about Sadie, about what it was—I mean, did you ever think there was one thing, one significant thing that made everything else weigh more heavily than it might have? Something that happened to her that you didn't know about, could never know about?" Luke stops talking, pauses, then says, "That makes no sense. I mean, something you perhaps didn't know about until later?"

The street is lushly dim with overgrowth, a pleached canopy of elm and eucalyptus. There is the silence of Louise's listening in the car, of her making sure that what has just been spoken has indeed been spoken. He feels reckless and he doesn't exactly want to feel that way, doesn't exactly not want to, either. He feels elated about Alice Samara, and then afraid to be, and then angry. The car dips into Louise's drive and he stops it abruptly.

"And why," Louise asks, "if I did know something, would I choose this moment, this time, to tell you?"

"Because I've finally asked," he says briskly, dangerously, because Louise will squash him for this flippancy. But then he pronounces the words again, point-blank, and very carefully . . . "because I have finally asked" . . . and he hears a sternness in his voice that has not previously been there in exchanges with her, and he hears the note of accusation, of offense he has taken and not till now allowed expression. He hears the sentence he spoke in the greenhouse, "This orchid is for my dead sister," hears the defiance in those words now. He didn't know he blamed Louise in any part for Sadie's death. He'd never felt anything but his mother and Sadie and himself against the world, against their father, against the medical establishment. But here it is, *blame*, explicitly inflecting his words—blame the most ineffectual response to any situation in existence. He feels horrified and he yanks the parking brake so deeply up into the tension of the car, he's not sure it will ever release. *The amount of experience you have in this field and you blame your mother—any mother—even unconsciously?* If his central nervous system verbalized itself right now, it would be hollering and sputtering at the same time—it would be comic, absurd.

"So what if you have finally asked," Louise says impatiently, looking out the window across her lawn. "Why would I ever have kept anything from you, Luke? Even if I'd wanted to, even if I'd felt guilty about something, responsible in a more drastic way than just the fact that I was her mother and she was my child and she died—how could I have kept anything from you as a doctor, a researcher?"

"I don't know," he says, angrily, "but maybe there's something so insignificant, you don't think it could have had any bearing, or something you've thought too crazy-sounding to ever mention?"

"Something really early on, you mean? It seems we discuss this every year—"

"Just talk about Sadie, Mom. Anything. Let's just talk about Sadie. Here. A restaurant. I don't care, but I want to hear more. I want to go over everything we've ever known or thought about or remembered. Did we have a dog ever?"

"This will help you? Or someone you're currently working with?" Louise asks, and he is about to say, Yes, yes it will, but she is no longer in the car, and Luke watches her through his windshield as she steps along the circular drive beneath the dense ficus trees to the kitchen entrance. If he didn't know her so well, he would detect no difference in her walk, but he does know his mother and he can see that her carriage is a little slower, heavier, as though she's pushing up against a medium already formed, one that she needs to find her way through and around. Luke feels remarkably angry watching his mother, and he's sorry his voice has relayed so much to her—to himself—brought so much back. He throws the locks, thinking to open all the doors, but then his shoulder hits up hard against the door as he tries to get out and he realizes he's locked himself in instead. He can't rid himself of these feelings of absurdity; smashing into his own car doors doesn't help. He throws the mechanism once again and getting out he hears very loudly his shoes against the gravel of the drive, and then the newspaper anchoring the orchids crunches sharply, and he hears the soprano of his mother's voice saying, "We never had a dog; Sadie was allergic"—all high-pitched sounds, shrieking in his ears in this moment to piercing. What's wrong with me? he thinks, and then the diagnostic mind in him suggests *auditory hyperactivity* as he hands two orchids to his mother, who is waiting behind him.

"Auditory hyperactivity," he says aloud, and he's struck by how low his voice sounds.

"Yes," his mother says slowly, gazing between the two plants in her hands, Sadie's orchid and another, "yes, I believe Sadie had that. I didn't understand that particular . . . affliction, I guess they called it, because at home she didn't keep her hands over her ears."

"And so what did you make of that?" Luke asks.

"That the world was too noisy—"

"No, I mean, did you argue with the doctors?"

"On that particular point?"

"Yes," Luke urges.

"I bought her earplugs, allowed her to wear them—you know all of this, Luke—and she heard everything through them. It wasn't that they deafened her, but they muted enough, the sounds of the classroom, traffic. It was hard for me to understand this as part of her schizophrenia—something physical in Sadie made her sensitive to sound. That didn't strike me as craziness, because the sounds that bothered her *were* horrible sounds, electronic sounds, high pitched, or incessantly whirring. It's not as though she was wrong. I wasn't going to gaslight my own child, tell her the cacophony out there was her fault."

"About thirty decibels of volume—"

"Enough. The plugs worked well enough," his mother says, turning and walking up the drive to the kitchen entry. Luke prongs three fingers into three plastic pots and grasps them in one hand. He's pretty sure his mother will not be happy with him for holding the orchids this way. He's almost forty years old and he still cannot take care! "The laziest kid God ever let live," his mother used to call him before Sadie died. It was actually twenty-nine decibels. He knows precisely the earplugs Sadie used to wear, the box they came in with the cardboard flap that read Quiet and then a big exclamation mark and then the word *please* uncapitalized but with an *r* in a small circle rising up from its ultimate *e*. Registered trademark, he supposes that meant, and he knows there's a difference between trademark and copyright, but he's not thinking about that so much now as he is about Sadie's

incredulous riff on the phrase *Quiet! please* as being somehow
something that a company could lay claim to. "It's totally weird,
Lukey Dukey, totally weird, when Mrs. Tornby says 'Quiet,
please.' I try to warn her, oh no, can't use that phrase, Mrs.
Tornby, they'll get you for that, little issue of a little r in a little
circle—ummm, ummm, ummm—makes a big issue, lots of dark-
minded men in dark suits, No, YOU be quiet, please! Mrs.
Tornby, it's true, ooops, they'll come for me, too. If they want you
to buy their product, care so much they own the phrase *Quiet!
please*, totally weird, 'cause who's saying that? It's an imperative,
you know—NO, what am I saying you don't know—IMPERATIVE,
LUKEY DUKEY!—a command, QUIET! PLEASE—shut up! But
who's saying that, and why would they want anyone to shut up
if they want you to buy their stupid little bungs—ten pairs of
ivory-colored foam plugs, 'For Sleeping, Shooting, Working,
Travel and Studying'—SHOOTING, do you see that? Says right
there, 'For Sleeping, Shooting.' Quiet! please, I'm shooting! Or
no, no, maybe they mean that when someone has a gun and
they're shooting it, you waddle on up to them and suggest a little Quiet! Please? I mean, HUH? Lukey Dukey, HUH?"

She was exhausting. Luke sighs now, remembering, completely exhausting, and he will despise himself for the rest of his
days—Hakuna Matata—for ever giving in to that exhaustion,
for hating the contortions of her face in her immense angry
befuddlement, "Lukey Dukey," how he hated her sometimes,
and she was smarter, always smarter than he was. He *did not*
know what *imperative* meant, not till he closed himself in his
bedroom and pulled the dictionary down from its high shelf,
maniacally tossing the pages, the *k*'s, the *h*'s, so few *i*'s, she probably knew the entire entry for that letter—where the fuck *were*
the *i*'s? He had even found the *j*'s before his furious, trembling
fingers settled, impediment, impel, imperceptive, imperator,
imperative—and then he read without sense, too tired, too
angry, that combination always . . . and then she was dead.

"No matter what," he says to his mother as she takes the
plants from him and they enter the tiled kitchen. "No matter
what—it always ends with 'and then she was dead.'"

Louise looks at him closely in the bright kitchen light, that perfect old skin, the clear blue eyes seeing so clearly. He is willing every goddamn lachrymal duct he possesses to reverse itself, to gush out the back of his neck if they have to, but they unload down his face, a fucking venetian blind of tears, behind which he can see nothing.

"Ah, Christ Almighty," Luke says. He reaches for the drawer beneath the counter where the tissues are, a drawer filled with cheesecloth and parchment paper, neat stacks of dish towels and hand towels. He loves his mother's ordered and well-stocked house, the house that had been his grandfather's, and when he rises, he sees her five Herend cachepots lined up down the counter waiting for their plants. He knows the name of the china pattern as well as he knows his own name, Rothschild Bird, and he sees that he has picked for Sadie an orchid too small for one of these.

"Maybe that's our problem"—his mother sighs, making an attempt at humor—"we didn't call upon the Almighty a long time ago."

"The Father, Son, and Holy Ghost—I'm the only one you got left, Mom—the Son!" But Luke realizes she's not laughing; she's turning the small white orchid with green markings around on the tile counter, inspecting it, looking under its leaves. She pulls the plastic label stick up from the soil and reads it as though it were a thermometer.

"*Brassavola nodosa*," she says, pronouncing the words carefully, and Luke hears it as a diagnosis, a classification, rare, a species, never hybridized, the death they have between them never recessed by any more dominant event in their lives, Sadie, Dead, and then she was never dead *and never changed, either.*

How did she die? Alice Samara will ask him some time. How did she die? And he will have to answer her, as he has answered this question many times before, and yet he has always fabricated, claimed various accidents—surfing, a car crash, drowning—and usually, in the last few years, he has taken to answering *childhood leukemia.* So unassailable this last. Cause of death: *childhood leukemia,* the most occult death of all, and yet never even a question. He's come to learn that everyone knows what leukemia is, that it doesn't even take Luke the doc to pronounce, to explain; everyone knows it's uncontrollable blood, uncontrollable something. Leukocytes, isn't it? But before Luke discovered the ease of leukemia as an answer, there'd been some awkwardnesses, moments in which Louise had saved his ass before he even knew he was mired in tar, "Yes, a surfing accident," Louise agreed, "so Luke has told you," or "No, she was too young to drive, but she did anyway," and all his mother had ever said in protest was once, quietly, pruning the espaliered pear, she'd suggested Luke keep her abreast of the flavor of this week's calamity. He despised her in that moment for protecting him. He despised her more for not allowing him his share of responsibility in Sadie's death—a share that he guesses has never occurred to her, that he feels his know-it-all-ness about drugs, and his assurances to her in those years, what might be called bedside manner, kept her from acting on her instincts. In twenty-one years she has not seemed to surmise his feelings about Sadie's death, his role in it—her role in allowing him his role! She'd always said she understood how hard it was to explain to others. That's all, but this time there's a difference in the air, a difference she's insisting upon: You will tell Alice Samara the truth—*a* truth, he amends, or another truth, because, in fact, he has been telling a truth: leukemia, but they never heard in *leukemia* Luke's name and the vowel sounds of Sadie's, nor in the word *leukocytes* his name once again and *oh* and *site*. . . .

But this time, because Janey will have provided Alice with certain accurate details—his mother is right—this time Luke will need to answer something approximating what actually happened. This is perhaps the work he'd wanted Janey to do with Alice, the aboutness of him he had—he realizes it now— set her up to accomplish before his arrival that morning at the studio, a shorthand *for him*, because maybe he can't get through the immense undergrowth without breaking down or becoming someone he thinks he isn't anymore.

"Do you have another one of these?" Luke asks, pointing at the cachepots, "a smaller one maybe?"

"Not to worry, darling. At this age, one has everything! Or at least everything material," she adds, stepping past him into the pantry. "Why don't you reach it for me," she calls, and Luke follows her into the huge pantry with its tall glass-fronted cupboards. "There," she directs, pointing to a far corner on one of the top shelves, her bracelets singing, "you see, there's a pair," and Luke does see. "These are beautiful," he comments, reaching down and placing one into his mother's hands. "I don't think I've ever seen them." They are a bluish white porcelain with acanthus leaves curling down to make handles. "You want just one of them, yes?" he asks, though it is not a question really, and then Luke slides the tall cupboard door closed, its glass panes chiming quietly.

"Your father liked these," his mother says, and Luke starts a little at the mention of his father, and even more so at the information that his father had liked something in this house. How his mother and father had ever gotten together, let alone married, is one of the great mysteries to Luke. His father seemed to revile almost everything his mother loved, or at least knew and so clung to—he loved the primitive as much as she loved the refined—and Louise had been strong enough, or somehow set happily enough in her ways, that she could take him or leave him; she had her children, their children, and his long absences hadn't seemed to matter much to her. She had had her great love, she once said, both Sadie and Luke in the living room at the time, sitting before the big fireplace with is intricate andirons; she'd had someone with beautiful dark eyes and dark hair, and his elegant generosities had mattered to her, his elegant cool manners. She was a senator's daughter and she knew how to be treated well, knew how to be the center of a huge and beautiful wedding, but then he had left her, no reason, really, she thought, just other meadows to graze in, he'd had his fun with her. She'd been just twenty-six, her mother long dead and her father's need of her more significant than ever. "And I had money," she told Sadie and Luke, not a huge amount, but enough, and this house and a way of life I knew and felt obliged to for many reasons—good reasons, she said. Luke knows more stories about his mother's first husband than he does about his own father. This was one of the strange facts of Luke's life, or maybe he'd remembered more about this man than he had about his father. But it hadn't been for not asking, Sadie and Luke pestering her to tell them stories, How did you meet Dad? What kind of a car did Dad drive? But they were the questions of children, and Louise had known this, and had told them the only romantic stories she knew, had lived, and they involved the man before their father, whose name she would never tell them, as he was famous by then, and famously married, and there were things that children just didn't need to know. Of course, Luke knew now who it was who had been his mother's first husband, and he thought this man's famous wife a more beautiful version of Louise, strangely, another politician's daughter and well brought up and known for her extravagant parties. "That was perhaps my problem," Louise would say. "I knew how to fade to the background, knew it wasn't about me—I wasn't enough of a showstopper, and didn't really want to be."

And Luke had found out later, too, how his own parents had met, a series of fund-raising lectures for UCLA, and how languorous a courtship it had been, archaeology always in the way, this dig here, that dig there, and their father bent on making his career, Louise still primarily by her father's side, giving dinner parties, making sure the right gifts were bestowed, and in the right manner and at the right time, and the endless, particularly sensitive personal correspondence. "I am a woman of another era," she always said, "except don't confuse that with prudishness or snobbery or cluelessness! You would be wrong in thinking that." And in saying this, his mother's voice would sometimes fade into pensive quiet, and at other times would ring out strong and jolly.

Luke says now, watching his mother settle moss around the orchids in their china pots, "I always expect a phone call, someone saying that Dad's body's been found."

"Luke, he could just as easily have run off with some sweet native girl without enough English to question him or to tell him no. That's what I think happened. I really can't fathom him dead in a cave somewhere in the Yucatán—he knew caves—I can't, and don't be surprised if one day he tosses up seeking your pardon—or money; he'd want that for sure."

"Why would Dad need money?" Lukes asks. He had wanted earlier to talk about Sadie, and they had for a time, and he'd received a kind of ultimatum from Louise, but somehow now his father's vague and definite absence constituted the conversation.

"Greed has nothing to do with need. An obvious point," his mother says, but this doesn't make much sense to Luke. If his father had wanted money, why wouldn't he have stayed with Louise, or stayed in contact? Lapses of logic were not common with Louise, and Luke thinks to just leave this alone. His father had been a chaired professor; he wasn't exactly penniless, but there had also been something strange in that their joint accounts had been cleaned out just before he went missing. . . .

"Saturday," Luke says. "Next Saturday, right?" he says more adamantly, as though he has an entire week to rehearse a performance, an entire week to script words that will sufficiently convey how his sister died, and why.

"And blame me," his mother says, taking up Sadie's orchid, and just as deftly taking up the subject of Sadie's death, "blame me all you want if that will help you," she says over her shoulder as she leaves the kitchen, the words coming back to him from the wide-open hall leading upstairs.

Luke hears her words as though she were standing directly in front of him, speaking. He has always had good hearing, excellent hearing, but within a normal range, excellent. What would it have been like to live in Sadie's head, to hear all she heard, pandemonium—all her demons speaking at once—and the effort it must have taken for her to sort it all out, to be coherent, even some of the time.

"Hey, I remember you," the valet says, jokingly, taking Luke's keys. "You're that guy who likes to valet twice."

"What, you don't have a mother?" Luke asks him coolly.

"Not a problem, man," he says, "not a problem," but Luke doesn't meet his eyes, nor those of the young valet closing his mother's door—the young valet who just an hour before had been throwing punches into the air above the sidewalk.

"I'm sorry," he says to the hostess as they enter the restaurant. "I didn't call. I thought we'd be early enough." But now they aren't that early, and Luke starts to think of some other restaurants—Joe's on Abbot Kinney—before the hostess says "Follow me" without looking at him. He doesn't like this restaurant, but Louise does, the goofy porcelain dishes, the beaded napkin rings. It's all a little too "gotten up" for his taste, perhaps not exactly a ladies-who-lunch place, but almost, and with a bitchy primness that doesn't seem to bother Louise but that sets Luke's teeth on edge.

"Why do you like this place?" he asks after the hostess has gone, leaning across the table, whispering. "It feels like housewares at Neiman Marcus."

Louise looks at him and smiles. She picks up her napkin and shakes it out. She takes her time laying it across her lap, her bracelets chattering. Her face is calmly portentous. "Yes?" he says.

"Even Janey likes this place . . ." she replies slowly.

"Yes?" he says again, now amused. He opens the menu, then turns it over to find the wine list. Not a good sign, a one-pager. What a snob he is, but still, they live in California, for God's sake! It's not as though this state doesn't produce any wine.

"He is not only a wonderful bartender; he's just fine to look at."

Luke casts his head around, looking at the bar. "Him?" he asks, chucking his chin at the cut of beefcake holding a cocktail shaker high above his head, giving his deltoids the itty-bittiest workout. "Janey has the hots for him, or just you?" he asks. What a show Los Angeles was.

"We share . . . which is rather becoming in a young woman, don't you think?"

Luke laughs, and it seems a long time since he's laughed, and laughed with his mother, who can be great company and who is very funny at times. He doesn't remember hearing of Janey ever being attracted to someone, of her ever making mention of someone's looks—sexual mention—man or woman.

Is this true, he wonders, or has he just not been around for it? "How is Janey?" he asks. "I haven't seen her in awhile."

"She's fine, Luke, and it's better that she has this job. You know that."

He hold his hands up, a show of giving in, surrender—they have made their decisions without him. Fine, whatever. "Any sign of a boyfriend?" he asks. "A girlfriend, anything?"

"No. I guess she's still all ours that way, but I think it's fine. I really do. Neither of us knows what Janey saw before the age of fifteen—I'm not even sure we want to know—but there are maybe some hurdles there for her to get across. But she will; I have no doubt. She will. There's nothing at all wrong with her."

Luke nods his head, he knows. "Her time will come," his mother usually said. He turns and looks back at the barman. "So, I take it we're drinking cocktails tonight? Whiskey sours should you want more of that muscle action over there."

"Why not. I've always liked action, Luke, but maybe it's your turn? How long's it been anyway?"

A glass with four crayons sits on the table between the salt and pepper shakers. Their flat-topped points are brand-new, and Luke puts the menu in his lap and pulls out the green crayon in honor of Stan. He begins to draw the interior of the greenhouse at Zuma Canyon Orchids, flower stalks going right and left. He takes a purple crayon and draws himself as an elephant, squeezed between the tables, "Luke" written across one wide ear. He uses the green crayon again to draw an orchid aloft in his trunk and to color in the nails of one of his great round feet stepping on a samara, the "dry, hard, winged fruit, as in the ash, maple, and elm; a key fruit," Luke recites as he draws. "It can't be her real name," he says to his mother. "Samara—she has to have changed her name."

His mother looks particularly handsome in this gentle light as she watches him. "Winged fruit," she says, an accent on all three syllables. Her eyes are lively and happy; he can see that she loves the idea of this young woman having changed her name to mean winged fruit. He's not sure he loves it so much; it's so L.A., everything a play that can be struck—the past whiped from the stage. Maybe this is something he needs to learn. He knows he should take his mother out more, should pay more attention, but as he thinks this, he says, instead, "Maybe it is my turn. It's been a long time, a very long time, but I don't really want to talk about that, either," he adds, rueful, smiling. He draws samaras all over the white butcher paper with a brown crayon, a whirl of them around the elephant's head. "They look like pelvises, don't they, or Fallopian tubes."

"You grew up seeing those," his mother says. "The two elms in the back—those elms must be seventy or eighty years old now. My mother planted them when they built the house."

"I did, didn't I?" Luke says. "Grow up seeing samaras. I wouldn't have remembered that if you hadn't told me. How fucking selective our brains are."

"Sweetheart," his mother says quietly, "Sadie would be institutionalized by this time—a fact you know better than I. If she were alive. Obviously, I'm not saying it's better she died, but when fate steps in, then you get on with your life, which you have and you haven't—"

Fate steps in, the phrase, echoes in Luke's mind, and the image of Sadie putting her foot down, pulling it back up, putting it down, snapping it up, *fate steps in*, the little jig she did the night before she died.

"You were right," his mother says quietly across the table, "you were right to tell Alice Samara about Sadie's orchid."

"It's an orchid, Mother, which we get for my dead sister, and that's about it."

"Oh no," she says, "no. There was much more to you saying that than the imparting of information. Much more. But it's right, Luke, and about time."

"What do you eat here," he asks, hoarsely. He has put down the crayons and taken the menu up from his lap. There is printing down the long folds of stiff manila paper, but it blurs before him.

"I drink martinis," his mother says. "I eat gravlax. I look at the pulchritude," and because the waiter is there, Louise takes the menu from Luke's hands and orders for both of them.

"Gravlax," she says, "and two Ketel One martinis, up," and though Luke hasn't drunk a martini in years and if he's going to do so would like it dirty, he doesn't say a thing. His life is changing, turning, and he knows it, wants it . . .

Henry Lutins appears for his afternoon appointment, sadly, heavily, fourteen years old but as massive in affect as a drugged bear. He's not drugged and hasn't been since he was ten, but if it's not an antidepressant or a soporific that courses through his veins, it's some other densening agent, which, Luke observes, thickens as the years go on. If Luke weren't schooled another way, he might linger more on this idea of, say, mortar setting up, a medium coagulating. Science or no, he finds something valuable in analogy, some insight into a thing without the presumption of being the actual thing, its horrors.

"Your grandson seems to be building a thicker and thicker wall against all forms of communication, Mrs. Lutins. I'm sorry." And yes, she understands this; Luke's seen it in her eyes. Her grandson the mason, that's certainly the grandson she knows, brick by brick, the scrape of his trowel becoming dimmer and dimmer, the wall immense now and Henry behind it.

Henry's grandmother has known for years the difference between the fusiform gyrus and the inferior temporal gyrus, and what happens and what does not happen and when and even a certain degree of why, but all that science, its *Fantastic Voyage* specificity, can't exactly capture the edifice of the boy she's up against, whose doors and windows she's worked for years to open.

Henry's been a patient of Luke's since he began private practice, and though Luke's long ago called in the family and laid before them his worst fears, his failure really, Henry continues to come to him because one of the few times Henry ever evinced emotion, violence in fact, was when they'd tried to stop the sessions. Luke knows—or thinks he knows—it's some clock or pattern set in Henry, rather than any actual desire, but if he were sure about anything with Henry, he might have been more successful at treating him, and yet the idea of success is difficult for Luke, as "success" in treating autism is too usually the creation of a circus act, children who learn to balance on the rump of a horse. God help them should they decide to step off that horse's ass—to walk out of the ring.

Luke believes their behavior should be modified, of course, but must they continue to be a cipher to themselves? He supposes it's somewhat necessary if any sort of social responsiveness is to be fostered, and yet he fears they're made to subdue themselves into rigid social norms—a pleasant mediocrity—rather than into movement in a direction best for their abilities—of which these children often have many. In his experience, autistic children are already confused over why people are alarmed at their behavior. They don't understand what effect they have on those around them. If Luke were to explain to Henry that his actions hurt his mother's feelings, that Henry should do unto others as he would have them do unto him, Henry would have no idea what Luke was talking about. Luke's worked hard to find some passage in Henry that will take him to a source, a spring, some distinct ability that might foster a meaningfulness beyond or even within the disorder.

Now, as though Henry were on a slow continuous dolly from door to chair, he moves into the office and comes and sits down with neither preamble nor willfulness in the chair across from Luke's desk. "Henry, how are you today?" Luke asks.

Henry moves forward in the chair and with his shoulder gestures to Luke as though to say, Okay Doctor. What about you? The motion is not flippant or resentful, but Henry's round, absent face seems as though it's in another room, in an entirely different context, listening to a speaker Luke can't see or hear. Henry wears a nice shirt, plaid, perhaps linen, cream and tan, a windowpane of red giving it sight lines, crosshairs. It puddles in Henry's lap, untucked, rather elegant. How well Henry's taken care of matters to Luke, tempers a sadness in him over Henry's life, over what might be done with it. "That's a fine-looking shirt, Henry—fine-looking on you," Luke emphasizes. Henry moves forward again in his chair, and then heavily, distractedly drags his hand down his shirt as though he means to smooth it. The fabric tautens alarmingly; a button pings against the desk. Luke would dearly love to know whether Henry has heard Luke's compliment as that, a compliment on his appearance, and if Henry is proud. Or whether Henry likes the shirt, too, is communicating that, is saying this fabric, its pristine stiffness, feels good, that he feels good within it. Then Luke does what he often does with Henry: He reminds himself that his thought processes aren't remotely close to Henry's, reminds himself once again that Henry's manifesting his fury in the mildest way he can. Or it might not even be fury this time, it might be the hair-trigger sensitivity some autistics have to touch, this tex- tured linen rough against his skin, but rough of a higher order, a rough that slams his nerve endings up against electricity.

"Take it off, Henry, if it doesn't feel good. Put it aside for the hour. Skins, okay. Know that expression? Skins? We usually have shirts on—and we should have shirts on—" Luke empha- sizes, "but today, hey, skins." Henry fingers his shirt buttons through their holes less slowly than Luke would have guessed, but no buttons fly. "Tell me what 'skins or shirts' means, Henry?" he asks, but Luke doesn't like what he hears himself saying. He's not being careful: the question is for an idiot, or at best a small child.

"Basketball," Henry says almost inaudibly. "In the street." He adds the word, *park*, but it falls from his lips like a scarf drifting of its own accord from a shoulder, event without cognition.

"Ever pick up a game? Go to the park, take a ball?" Luke asks. He looks at Henry's bare chest, which is broad and muscu- lar, a chest more adult than Luke expected, not the chest of a patient as inanimate as Henry, nor as adolescent. Luke imagines Henry flanking a lithe center, rising from his feet for a shot, Henry a huge and graceful guard. It's not a paternal thought, Luke the surrogate father dreaming his son into prowess, so much as a curiosity about Henry's physical abilities. The careful

alacrity with which Henry divested himself of his shirt compels
Luke, and he asks, "Handle a ball? Dribble? Run? Can you shoot?
Man, Henry, you never told me you played basketball."

Luke watches complete incomprehension register on
Henry's face, though *register*, he notes, is too strong a verb—as
is the word *complete*. Henry doesn't understand because now,
without transition, Henry's in that other room, attending that
other voice, the lecture only Henry can hear. What Luke has
tried for years to find for Henry is focus, some discipline or
craft upon which the intensity of his autistic mind might fixate
productively. For a time, Luke thought it might be music, as
once, in the outer office, and years ago, Henry had refused to
budge from his chair, to come into Luke's office, when always
before, and ever after, Henry moved where he was asked to
move. *Prayers of Kierkegaard* played on the radio, but Luke had
had to ask Albertine to call the station to find that out. She
reached first to turn up the sound, and Luke could see that
Henry deepened in his responsiveness to the mounting liturgi-
cal chant. Albertine spoke quietly into the telephone and then
wrote "*Prayers of Kierkegaard*" on a pad of paper, "Opus 30, by
Samuel Barber," and handed it across her desk, but Luke was
already somewhere else, thinking about music and Henry, and
music and autism in general, and this recurring line in the
Barber, "O Thou who art unchangeable," or was it "O Thou
who art unchanging"?

Luke thinks about this day every time he sees Henry, thinks
of this chanted sentence or praise, this great human hunger for
constancy, something known and powerful and abiding. God as
autistic is not a new thought for Luke, nor thoughts of the
immense powerfulness of autistic children to maintain their
omniscience against the world, God-ing themselves, but Henry,
bare-chested before him, is not benign, and he is not all-
powerful; he is not wrathful, not full of fury and command-
ment, nor is he beneficent and charitable and kind. He is not
even particularly disappointed. What is Henry? Luke asks himself now. He who art unchanging, and if he, Luke, cedes Henry
power, if he, Luke, configures this immense ability of distrac-

tion as just that, *ability*, then Luke holds to a shred of free will within Henry; stupidly, against all intelligence, Luke has held to the idea of ability. And finally that ability has been found, even though years ago Luke had tried to throw in the towel.

Luke has stood between Henry and an institution, and on this issue, Luke's not conflicted. By Henry's age, most children with his problems have been institutionalized, maybe for some time, but Henry has a grandmother who will hear none of this, who will pay Luke almost any amount of money to keep her grandson at home. Many autistic children belong in institutions, Luke is sober-minded about this, but he surmises that Henry, away from home, would worsen even further, and away from faces that may manifest in his brain differently than they do in psychotypical children's brains, but manifest they do nonetheless, even if there have been many, many times in which Henry did not recognize his own mother.

Luke's had a hard time reading Henry's parents, what they may wish for their son, whether Henry in their life is how it is and they embrace him and life goes on, or whether Henry's autism stopped their lives cold. There are religious convictions, too, and a profound sense that you do not send away your own. But what Henry's parents may wish is so shrouded by the grandmother's financial and religious authority, Luke can't ascertain whether she's welcome guidance, financial security, or whether she's a colossus of judgment who blocks their desires, catches them like arrows and chucks them away.

Luke's aided the grandmother and he doesn't know whether this is good or bad, doesn't know what he's wreaked in the lives of Henry's parents. He's good for Henry—that he supposes to be true—and he's good for the grandmother's sense of hope, but Luke harbors a sheepish sense of having helped forestall Henry's parents not only from other children but from a life of their own, away from the husband's mother, her insistent righteous presence as the primary caretaker of Henry. Luke likes old Mrs. Lutins, the heavy German pocket watch she wears around her neck on a chain of gold matrix and bloodstone, her alligator pocketbook and matching pumps. She steps down from celluloid every time he sees her, every time he hears the Hitchcockian anticipation of her heel taps across his outer office floor. She's a woman who knows how to walk in heels, to move, an old-world elegance, but there is the Moral Monster about her, too. He has no doubts that she can toss across the holiday table observations so intricately damning, there's no defense against them short of fleeing. In fact, Luke knows from an early interview with Henry's mother that her prenatal diet—that teratogenic smorgasbord she gorged herself upon—is something referred to more than occasionally by old Mrs. Lutins. "Chocolate? Salami? could these have had an effect?" Henry's mother had pleaded with Luke: Prosciutto? the glass of champagne at her sister's wedding she'd sipped happily in her third trimester, its pernicious alcohol? No doubt she'd eaten fish sodden with mercury and vegetables gorgeous from pesticides!

But no, Luke had assured her from across his desk, no, calming her. "And anyway, you didn't eat any salami or prosciutto, did you, Rahel?" he'd asked, thinking to bring her back from the edge of hysteria, to remind her of who she was. He remembered watching her shake her head of thick black curls, first one way—no, she'd eaten no salami, no prosciutto—and then the curls going the other direction more slowly, then rapidly, all curls—he couldn't see her face—yes, she had, deliberately, against all interdiction, religious, medical, the curls frantically affirmative, a plate of melon sheathed in translucent trichinous flesh. Luke thought all of Italy might be morons or autistics if prosciutto presented the dangers suggested, but he'd not said that, had made instead the professional comment that cured meats—if improperly cured—could . . . but it was no use thinking about all of this now, with Henry before him, Henry the result of those nine happy months, trouble-free, easy; that had been the word Rahel Lutins had used: "Easy—it was an *easy* pregnancy!" Then there was Henry, sweet, docile Henry, but after a time distracted Henry, then inattentive and clumsy Henry—oh so clumsy—and finally—though it was just the beginning—absent Henry in all his presence, like living with a child sculpted of butter . . . "like living with a goddamned ham," Rahel Lutins had screamed in his office years ago.

Henry moves unselfconsciously in front of Luke, a bear getting comfortable in a chair, a chair a little too small, a little too hard—a bear who doesn't know someone has shaved him of a great patch of fur, though, of course, it is just his shirt that is doffed, Luke thinks, just that patch missing. "How's your job, Henry?" he asks.

"People have questions, and they don't know," Henry says solemnly.

"What do they ask you?"

"You know," he says.

"And you answer their questions."

"Lacunae," Henry says.

"In their knowledge or in the information given for the exhibits?"

Henry shakes his head. He's in the other room, attending the other lecture. Luke waits several beats. Albertine drops something flat and heavy. It slaps loudly against the tile of the front office. Luke hears her murmur something—or actually, what Albertine says is a murmur by the time it reaches him. "Henry," says Luke, calling him back, firmly, quietly. "Henry, explain to me what you mean by 'lacunae.' Where? In whose knowledge?"

"Yeah, well," he says. "They don't know that."

It's long not surprised Luke that Henry uses words like *lacunae*. Oddly, wonderfully, the man who'd hired Henry to work in his small museum was not ever surprised—as far as Luke knows—by Henry's vocabulary. Luke adores that fact. "I assume there's something wrong with the kid?" the man had asked gruffly. "That's why you're here?" Luke had hesitated a long time, had gazed about the small dark foyer before the entrance of shabby maroon drappery leading to the displays and tanks, smelling the tang of salt water mingled with the must of the museum and the man himself, unbathed for perhaps four or five days. "Likes my lobsters instead of broads—of course there's something wrong with him," the man said, downcast.

"But he knows a fuckload about crustaceans, I'll say that for him. Excuse my language, Doctor."

"Where do you think he learned it?" Luke asked, turning around to look at the man's pinched blue face. It was the black light and the heavy stubble, and perhaps some ability learned from his marine charges of living with less oxygen. "Did you teach it to him?"

"I see you're one of those fancy people," the man said, "—think they can teach someone something. I didn't teach him jack."

Are you going to teach him Jill, though? Luke thought to himself, because instananeously every intuitive hackle on his body was up and alert and signaling. Something flew off this man that Luke didn't like, and it had nothing to do with his shabbiness, but, rather, his ready defensiveness within the context of teaching. Something *anti*-moralistic, as though Luke had suggested he nail up the Decalogue or something, make museumgoers recite it devoutly before proceeding to view crayfish and crabs and krill. Luke wasn't particularly righteous, but he was dead willing to announce where the stops were. You might not have taught Henry anything, he thought, but will you allow him any inclination he has? Are you the type of "sage" who will watch a baby reach into a fire because, hey, they won't do *that* twice—or they will and that's all the better for you? If Henry rubs himself up against a chair or a table, will you offer him a glory hole?

"The kid's a nutcase," Luke said, feeling mean, acting it, not wanting Henry a part of this quirky enterprise, as accepting as it was of him. "Henry's autis—"

"No, he ain't," the man retorted quickly.

Luke had been through interviews like this before, the ready refusal of a patient's illness, of Luke's expertise. Not denial exactly—that constituted a different group of responses—but this refusal—and those of its ilk—insisted on a higher level of intelligence about the patient, unequivocal evidence, the "Prove to me that isn't just eccentric behavior" response. Every Tom, Dick, and Harry was a psychotherapist these days.

"He is, I am," the man said, but now his voice softened, deepened down into something blustery, but mostly morose, despondent. Luke could love the man for his defense, would have —years ago, a teenager—joined him, passed the good bong— "Society, yeah, too fucking uptight, man"—but now Luke knew degrees of behavior better than most, imagined Henry grasping an aquarium too tightly, the shards bleeding him into shock before he even noticed his shirt heavy, wet with blood, as dark a color as the museum's strange massive drapery. He could imagine Henry startled into hysteria by the scrape of a lobster claw, even the gentle electrical static of someone's arm hair across his own. What Luke couldn't imagine was that this would all go well, would be all right, hunky-dory, copacetic. He couldn't imagine that this would not end badly, dangerously so. And then there was this issue of a sexual education, and of sexual predation, of which the mentally ill were especially vulnerable, especially someone like Henry, who was bereft of any ability to read intention, good, bad, indifferent. And where Henry was in the sexual fun house was a mystery to Luke, to his grandmother and parents. Masturbation, even the beginnings of genital exploration? Henry didn't even seem to be looking at himself in the funny wavy mirrors. Luke had waited to see if sexual activity didn't effect a change in Henry, some livening of the circuitry. There'd been nary a spark.

"If you give him a routine, you can't vary it," Luke stated adamantly. "In fact, you need to give him a routine, very definite, very established."

"What might happen?" the man asked, serious now, his words charged only with concern. Luke wanted to say to him, I understand your defense of him stems in great part from a defense of your own strangeness, but Henry Lutins is unpredictable and perhaps more powerful than he is physically because of that unpredictability. What Luke said was, "He presents a variation of a condition called Asperger's disorder," and Luke had explained to the man as much as he knew about Henry Lutins, divulging to the brink of confidentiality. "He seems docile, and for the most part he is, but I've seen him otherwise."

"Okay, sure," the man agreed, "and he takes the bus to you on Tuesdays and Thursdays."

"You always play classical music?" Luke asked, getting ready to leave; he'd had a full day of patients, and then the sprint down Venice Boulevard to this small brick building slung with fishing nets and plastic crabs, Museum of Crustaceanna. "Henry's particularly fond of a Samuel Barber piece called *Prayers of Kierkegaard*, Opus Thirty."

"How many years you been treating Henry and you don't know he knows about this stuff?"

He's Jewish; he's not supposed to know anything about shellfish, Luke wanted to say, to joke, but no, he had no idea Henry knew anything about crustacea. Luke pushed his card across the narrow counter. "I'd like to talk regularly, every couple of weeks. Please don't misread me. I'm delighted you've given Henry this chance, that you've encouraged him." Luke said this last, but he left uncomfortable, asking himself why acceptance seems so often in places of squalor or semi-squalor, the marginal, down-at-the-heels world?

Now Luke watches Henry closely. *Jill*, he keeps thinking, *Jill*. Is the guy up to anything? Has Henry been initiated in any way, even by verbal suggestion? But Henry seems unchanged. "I understand, Henry, that you're asked questions at the museum and that you answer them. Exhaustively. Why is it you won't answer my questions?"

Henry tips forward in the chair, his eyes focused on some corner of the room behind Luke. His head pivots one way, another; maybe there's some insect on his body somewhere but he can hardly place it. Or he might like the small quiver of its incremental progress. Luke thinks not, but who would know?

"Henry?" Luke says.

He moves again, lumberously, his head lolled back. "You might never have asked me anything about a crustacean?" he says.

"What if I really did want to know about flea shrimp or something, would you tell me, Henry?"

"Which *Daphnia* do you want to know about? There are hundreds at the museum. Which one?"

Classic, Luke thinks, "Which one?" and indeed Henry does mean, "Which one?" Weak central coherence. "Do you have one you think is of particular note?"

"No. I note them all," Henry says with no self-consciousness, with the absence of affect that is usual with him. Long ago, Luke observed that Henry, though bearlike, also had the slow-witted, heavily undulant quality of life under water. Now he emulates this quality even more acutely, perhaps because now he spends hours surrounded by slowly bubbling aquariums, blue and cold and emotionless. Had something finally been found for Henry? Luke fears they've secured his seclusion.

"Tell me about crustacean endocrinology?"

"B. Hanström is responsible for the discovery of the X-organ in crustaceans. This organ, together with the related sinus gland, constitutes an anotomic complex that has proved of great interest in understanding crustacean endrocrinology. One view holds that neurosecretory cells in the X-organ and the brain produce a molt-preventing hormone that is stored in the sinus gland of the eyestalk; other theories postulate a molt-accelerating hormone produced in a Y-organ. The interrelations of these two hormones may be responsible for the molting process."

"Thank you, Henry."

Luke's now become the Sino-espionage doctor practicing hypnosis in *The Manchurian Candidate*, thanking—dispatching—the subject after he's performed perfectly according to the evil plan. Or he's the ringmaster center ring he's fought so hard not to be. *You will now observe Henry perform the difficult stunt of balancing on the rump of a moving horse as he attempts to shake hands with Albert, our master clown.* Henry rises slowly and turns to walk to the door. His shirt remains draped across the chair arm. Luke reminds him he needs to reclothe himself and Henry does so without argument, even seemingly without hearing Luke's instruction. Henry fingers the buttons nimbly, no longer a child with severe motor-control problems. There's been some success, some, but as Henry nears the hole missing its button, Luke senses the need to circumvent an episode. Luke walks from behind his desk and falls to his hands and knees, pulling his hand across the carpeting, trolling for the button Henry's popped from his shirt. "You're missing a button, Henry. Let me find it for you. I bet someone at home will sew it back on for you." The button might be swallowed by any number of his patients, and this alone insists the button be found, but Henry is also made anxious by disturbed series, and looking up, Luke can see the panic setting into Henry's face, and though it's a mild panic, it's not one Luke wants to have to explain. "It's okay, man, we'll find this button," and just then Luke's hand feels the small smoothness between his fingers.

He pushes a halting grocery cart through Gelson's, leaning against it on the right in order to keep it on course, wishes they'd *stop fucking waxing* the apples and oil their carts. He likes the idea of cooking for Alice, of putting food on a table and watching her face. He wants it to be summer, a better time of year for tomatoes and peaches, not that he can't actually buy tomatoes now, and even apricots and peaches; they're here beautifully displayed, but waxen-looking, too perfect, as though no bug would deign to eat them. What does *she* deign to eat? Luke wonders, but he knows trauma is not there for her, is not in food or vegetation or flowers. He has thought to find in her life what went wrong, the catastrophic, but he's weary of those thoughts right now, understands them to be less about Alice than about what has happened to Alice, that there is a distinction and that locating trauma serves his profession but not his heart. He chooses five slender Persian cucumbers hardly the length of his hand and he knows she'll like these, sliced to coins, tossed with shallots, chervil fronds, French olive oil. Of course, he does not know for certain that she'll like them—

Stan Mingis's father is leaning over the lettuces. Luke watches him shake water from a small bunch of red leaf, then put it down and take up a head of romaine. Seeing people out-side the context of the office is always difficult, sometimes even significantly disturbing.

"Doctor," Mr. Mingis says as Luke approaches, *Doctor*, an acknowledgment but not a salutation. Luke has learned not to appraise parents from these chance moments, that doing so cashes them all in as defensive, cold, forbearing, pretty much denominations they're not, though certainly they've had to learn forbearance whether they wanted to or not—having an autistic child is under *forbearance* in the dictionary.

"How are you, Mr. Mingis?" Luke asks. "Any lettuce worth being peeled for?"

Mr. Mingis gives a shrug. He might actually be trying to laugh, Luke thinks, might actually be trying to say, Ah well, you know how shopping at Gelson's is. But then Mr. Mingis reaches up and rips a plastic bag from the roll and says, "I'm fine, Doctor; it's my son, of course, who's sick."

Luke knows to touch upon something parents can do, something they take control of and do well. "You got great taste in film," Luke says, an intentional vernacular in his syntax, and finally Mr. Mingis does laugh, quietly, resignedly as he tucks the romaine stem down into the clear plastic. Luke watches how gentle he is, that he doesn't jam it or stuff it, that he works the thin plastic sheath up the long leaves.

"I don't know about *The Lion King*," Mr. Mingis says. "I'm not sure I rank that up there with *The Manchurian Candidate*. I live in horror of him seeing something like *Aliens III*—every other word would be *fuck*."

Luke tugs his cart out of the way of other shoppers. He reaches for oak leaf, watercress, miner's grass. "Actually," he starts to say to Mr. Mingis, "actually," he says again, "the *Alien* scripts aren't linguistically complex enough for Stan—he'd be uninterested in them."

Mr. Mingis turns and looks seriously at Luke. He's tall and very tan and yet, Luke observes, there's no health in the tan, it's as though it's makeup. It's been a long time since they have spo-ken, and this is the recognition coming into Mr. Mingis's face.

"You play tennis, don't you, Doctor?" Mr. Mingis asks. "Perhaps we could grab some time tomorrow, talk a bit. I realize we—"

"Great," Luke says. His ability at tennis is splendidly abysmal and the last activity in the world right now he wants to pursue is tennis, but if Mingis will talk, Luke will chase down his line drives till Halloween.

"I think I live in terror of him, Doctor."

"You're brave enough to play tennis with me," Luke says, smiling. "We'll talk tomorrow. Early would be better."

"Sure," Mr. Mingis says, "sure thing. I'll call your office."

Luke watches the gabardine of Mingis's suit move fluidly about his legs as he pushes his cart down the aisle. It's a beautiful suit, as though the fabric has lead or water threads in its weave, an undulant, dramatic weight that makes it enfold and unfold as Mingis moves. Luke can never bring himself to pay that kind of money, but he thinks, maybe some day? Maybe to marry Alice in—but he punts the thought from his head. What has made him want her so suddenly, without question or pause, and want her with permanence, assurance, some guarantee no matter how delusional? He scares himself, this careering—even vicariously—into images of a future not really very much in his control. Why don't you see if she likes your cooking, asshole? The red potatoes feel smooth and heavy in his fingers, a serious coldness within their skins. He counts sixteen into a plastic bag, and then watches one tumble out across the floor, then another and another, the rent in the seam of the bag opening farther as more and more plummet, till they are all free and bobbling about amid shopping-cart wheels and the shoes of shoppers.

Someone is on his way immediately to help, popping potatoes into the marsupial pocket of his apron as he approaches.

"Not to worry, sir," he says. "Just select yourself some more. I'll get these."

Luke stoops to pick up a potato near him and catches sight of Mr. Mingis down the aisle looking back at him, an expression of pain on his face, trying to be amused. Luke waves the potato sheepishly, and yet he wants to rise and wind up and pitch it at his head, knock from Mingis's senses any notion that his competency as a doctor is reflected in grocery store foibles. Luke wishes to hell he played tennis better, knows Mingis sees himself shagging balls for most of their game tomorrow. What assholes we all are, Luke thinks, and wonders, *Why?* Is there always this much intricate nastiness among people? Among men? He straightens up, knows he has a nostalgia for something that absolutely never existed, a simplicity within masculine exchange that probably happens more today—if at all— than it ever did. Once again, the potatoes feel cold and smooth in his fingers, like a museum floor, he thinks, and then he realizes the plastic bag is heavy, that he has forgotten to count, and holding the bag up before his eyes he gauges he has enough potatoes for ten Alices, maybe eleven. He can feed her reflection refracted many times. What a fanciful thought, a long line of Alices in the mirror of his entry hall, and he is standing behind her, holding her firmly there within the quicksilver.

"Industrial, mechanical, clinical, pathological—who has taken flowers in these directions?" Alice Samara says to him on the tile and brick patio of his mother's house. She laughs, teasing herself. "Oh, sure, there's always been the automotive direction, tires used as planters, hubcaps outlining a flower bed, but I find in most ways flowers have been left in the nineteenth century, which may be why they comfort us so, or taken back to ninth-century Japan—both amazing, but ultimately nostalgic, and I think that's the one thing flowers teach us not to be, nostalgic."

He still doesn't know whether she's fascinating, brilliant, or a crackpot. He hands her a Scotch, neat, off his mother's tea cart. He likes the way she holds her glass, her hand dropped down by her side, the glass suspended loosely between thumb and middle fingers, almost as though the glass is a bucket suspended from the bail of her fingers.

"Pathological," he says to her back. "I guess I don't under-stand how—or what—that would be."

"Florally speaking," he then says to himself quietly.

She stands, looking out over the yard. She doesn't turn to face him. "It's really not the right word," she says, and he doesn't know whether she's heard him mutter "florally speaking" under his breath and is just not defensive, or whether she's in fact checked herself. She pulls her glass up to her lips and drinks, and he watches the fabric of her blouse pull across her back, tiny rows of gathered silk, and then as her arm drops, the fabric sheers again, just one thin layer beneath which her lingerie appears. He wonders where Janey is, as she is supposed to be here by now too, Janey, the Gilded Thistle, he thinks. When Janey arrives, some-thing will be explained, satisfied; she'll be a rubric for the evening, a guide to Alice. Of this he assures himself. What he doesn't understand already is Alice's ease, loquacious, for Christ's sake, and the clothing she wears, which is expressly formal, the silken blouse and the blue velvet lounging pants. He's sure the word *barbecue* characterized his mother's invitation, barbecue in the garden, code for casual, but Alice had appeared at the door, several small packages in her hands, a minuscule embroidered purse suspended from her wrist, a wrist that he noted was not scarred, either across or lengthwise, though why he expected it to be bothers him. He had helped her settle the several little boxes onto the entryway table, and then she had turned and said, "What a beautiful old house—what amazing tile work."

Now she is saying, "You know the grass that grows on the freeway? Along where the roadbed ends and the shoulder begins—that narrow corridor of grass that sometimes goes on for miles. I'm always interested in that when I drive. It seems immensely hopeful—the natural world reclaiming itself."

Of course you're interested, he feels compelled to answer, though does not. She has walked farther down into the yard, down the bricked steps and into the lower terrace. Of course she finds vegetation within the endless concrete desolation of the Los Angeles freeways, of course. He is intensely sure that were she stripped of all her resources, she would still find some muscular seedling hefting the earth on its shoulders in order to sprout. Why? he wants to know, his attraction to her as diagnostic as it is sexual. Why? He sees her move deeply into a forest; she's a sturdy-limbed little girl with long hair falling down around her shoulders and arms. She knows where she's going; the terror is behind her, farther and farther behind her, the forest darkening in protection, in verdancy, in calm.

"I like also when you see that someone has planted something in a can," she calls to him as though confiding. "It's on a stoop or a window ledge; there can be trash all around, poverty, but there is this cup of dirt in a soup can and a sprig of mint or chive having a life—I like that a lot, too." Luke supposes these confidences would seem strange to most people, that she could not sit through a date with just anyone and tell these things.

"I guess Alice didn't feel she could bring flowers," his mother comments as she emerges through the French doors at the back of the house. Within her arms are all the small packages Alice Samara has brought. Luke likes his mother, has always liked her, even when he was a teenager, found her reasonable, funny, her comfortable elegance soothing, and he thinks this now, how much he likes his mother. Whatever is in each package, she'll find its appeal. "Hey," he says to his mother, "hey, we've got a samara in the yard!" and they both laugh. "Except it's the wrong season." Then Luke whispers, "You ask her," and Louise says, "No, you ask her."

"Ask me what?" Alice says as she walks back up from the yard, her drink moving at her side. Luke watches her quick, swift carriage. She has the appeal of something viewed through a microscope, an alert, edgy movement whose quickness alone rivets attention—though one is never quite sure one has seen it, that it's ever been there, meant what one thinks it might mean. "I would normally bring flowers," she says, going on. "Without apology I would, but it seemed unimaginative in this case—do those flowering maple last for any amount of time in water?" she asks, statement and question running into each other, a habit of conversation she has that interests him. "Their stems arch so perfectly," she adds.

"Not long enough," comes from inside the house, the words funny and snide and pronounced with full awareness of how they will play. Janey appears in the doorway holding in each hand a bottle twisted about with brown paper bagging. "Swill," she announces, holding the bottles up triumphantly, "glad to be invited." She plunks the bottles down on the table and, when they totter, grabs them up again and takes them back through the doors into the kitchen. Brogans, pedal push-ers, a vintage shirt of some mad scientist's alchemical thread— Janey's usual palette of clothes, Luke notes, a wardrobe archly between destitute and enervated high fashion. And hair the color of antifreeze! "What are you drinking?" he asks her as she reappears.

"Scotch. Like the boss."

He thinks it interesting that though Janey dresses unusu-ally, like an artist, say, or someone young, innovative, it's not Janey who's the fabulist. He pours Janey's Scotch and then holds an ice cube poised over the glass as he hands it to her.

"Oh, yeah, ice, please," Janey says, relieved, and he loves Janey for her willingness to be both uncomplicated and some-one who gasps, "enough already, give me something *I* want." He's never known Janey to drink Scotch before, and though he chides himself on the incredible immaturity of it, he still wants Janey to be employed by his family, his mother, for Janey's attentions to be in the service of this garden and house. He still wants Janey to be theirs alone. Louise had been healthier about it than he had, he supposes, pushing Janey out on her own. "Two bad marriages and a dead child is not work that someone else should have to shoulder," his mother had said, but still this annoys Luke. He doesn't see exactly how the past must control who Janey is to them, for them. "How can I ever pay Janey enough for making me happy in the way Sadie made me happy? How can I arrive at a conscionable salary for such a service?" He hears it all again in his head, hears "I can't love Janey like I loved Sadie. It's not fair to Janey, the contrast, and she's a sorry comparison to Sadie, who's practically mythic, for Christ's sake. I wish it were Janey who was dead."

Luke is watching his mother hug Janey now in the yard, in front of Alice. He can't see on his mother's face anything but relief that Janey stands within her grasp, and then her arms straighten, pushing Janey out before her, turning her around. "God, the way this kid dresses. It's pure artistry."

"What's for dinner, Geez Louise?" Janey asks. Alice walks back into the garden, leaving them all. She is at the farthest reach, along the brick wall. Luke watches her do something rather striking. She carefully places her Scotch glass on her head and walks the entire width of the back wall, which is espaliered with three fruit trees, a pear, an apple and a clementine. She passes in front of the branches trained to point up the wall like tridents, the glass riding perfectly still atop her head, and he watches her make a tight, careful turn and glide back in the direction she has just come.

"You see your boss now?" he asks Janey, pointing down the garden, but when she looks, Alice is striding toward them, her glass once again in the bail of her fingers at her side.

"Yes," Janey says quizzically, and he is forced to dissemble, to stammer out that Alice seems to be at home, to like the garden, to have found inner peace, for God's sake. Janey laughs, and though she's not seen the finishing-school performance at the end of the garden, she is certainly aware of the possibilities within the arena called Alice. She casts a bemused look at Luke and he smirks at her, a ha-ha look on his face—they might as well be brother and sister.

"I want to see what all Alice has brought you, Mother," he says. "Let's sit down a bit."

A flower frog in the shape of a turtle appears from a wrapping, and he figures it to be quite old, and perhaps Japanese, something he thinks just as his mother says it. It's a singular little piece and he can see that Louise likes it immediately. The three women talk about Ikebana, the different schools, he hears moribana, shofu, seika, several reverential comments about their teachers; he hears the names Mrs. Saneto, Mr. Matsumoto, a discussion of bases, rocks, kenzan. He's ignorant of this entire discipline, but he's happy listening. The little toasts his mother has made sit undisturbed on a side table. He supposes he might get up and fetch the tray and walk around the table, munching from it. He knows they would all laugh, that he would present an image of maleness to them which completely satisfies some heartfelt definition they harbor. His mother unwraps a particularly tiny book, so tiny that he cannot make out its subject matter, held as it is within her fingers. He keeps meaning to push himself out of his chair to retrieve the hors d'oeuvres, but Alice sits so that the breeze carries her scent and settles it on him like a net. He does not move, cannot remember the command within his circuitry that might goad his legs into standing. The little book is erotica and he's amused—perhaps even a little amazed—that Alice had the nerve to give it to his mother, though of course Janey would have schooled her: "Louise is a broad, you don't have to watch every word or stay clear of any subject that matters in life." Luke can just hear Janey getting up a head of steam over the state of what she called, in her parlance, discourse; he could hear her telling Alice that Louise would start to get bored pretty quickly if sex wasn't part of the discussion, or religion or politics. "Louise will talk food and flowers for a time—they're de rigueur—but she'll insist they can't carry an evening." Luke, listening to Janey in his head, laughs out loud—Janey and Louise might as well be mother and daughter. The table stops and all three women turn to look at him.

"No, no," he stammers, "I was laughing about what Janey would have told Alice about old Louise here. I wasn't—" he starts to say, but then realizes the little toasts await him, mercifully, and he rises quickly and retrieves the tray and starts to pass them. "Smoked trout, I presume," he says jokingly. "Itty-bitty bits of smoked trout."

"I've always loved this Teraoka painting," Louise says. "That's one happy woman—"

"More like one happy octopus," Luke says, seeing the painting in miniature over his mother's shoulder, the great languid squid between the tattooed woman's legs, the look of ecstasy on both their faces.

"They translate the inscription," Alice says, and Louise reads, "'A woman sunbathing at the beach and while sleeping a sliminess comes over her body. "Is this my suntan lotion that feels so good?" she says. "Hmm."'"

"So, you know his work?" Alice asks Louise as their delight subsides, but Luke does not hear his mother's answer because the timer is buzzing on the oven. He walks through the doors, across the tiled breakfast room, and into the kitchen. He realizes he's still carrying the tray of toasts. For a silly instant, he stands trying to decide whether to carry the tray back out to the patio or whether to just set it down here while he bastes the chicken. He bristles at himself, his indecisiveness, the magnificently minor nature of his deliberation. But it's Alice, and he's giddy with her, the thought of her. Worse than having the hors d'oeuvres where no one can sample them is the four or five minutes he'll not hear her voice and words, her comments, and though usually he likes plunging the baster into the hot oils, watching them mount solidly in the tube, and then squeezing them out over the glistening bird, now he's fussed by having to do it. He peers through the oven door, sees the chicken skin still has a pale suppleness, and returns to the patio. As he settles the tray down on the table, he sees again the ferny lace beneath the silk of Alice's blouse, and he sees that she hardly fills the chair, that she sits poised like an apple on an otherwise-empty surface. And though he does not want to use the word, it springs to his mind, *encapsulated*, the meaning of that diagnosis within his discipline, though she's not, he knows, not encapsulated in any pathological sense, but, rather, in what he sees as a lack of differentiation between the conscious and the unconscious in her work. There was a wedding picture in the book, and he wants to say to her now, What did you mean by such an arrangement? He realizes in this moment—not earlier with the book actually before him, but now, looking at Alice sitting half on the chair and half on some plane of her own body's making—that the flowers are all *behind* the bride, cascading from her veil, from the crown of her head, from her cheeks and shoulders and hips, lilacs and roses separating from her as she emerges, her hands held simply before her, gathered within themselves. Luke finds the simplicity of the hands incredibly vulnerable and incredibly powerful at the same time, and the bride's face, as though from beneath the ground the face and hands are a spring, a source, the promise water is—that simple, that powerful.

Alice Samara trusts what her hands can do, he thinks to himself; she trusts what she makes. And it's an interesting verb, because he doesn't feel that she trusts much.

Janey is telling the story of Louise and the 7-Eleven clerk, Janey waiting and waiting in the car for Louise, who has only just popped in for some cream, Janey parked to the side of the store, ping-ponging through a magazine, waiting, caught up ultimately in an article about vegetable hair dyes, but waiting, wondering, What on earth? and then finally a quarter of an hour later, Janey getting out of the car and walking to the front of the store just in time to see the store clerk throwing his arms around Louise and hugging her, covering her face in kisses. "Like he's a goddamn Labrador gleeful at the appearance of his mistress," Janey says.

"I couldn't leave the clerk in there alone. The guy was obviously about to hold him up, was waiting for me to leave."

"So you just waited him out?" Alice asks. She laughs a little wonderously.

"I could see the gun at the back of the guy's jacket when he leaned over to pick up a magazine. And I could just feel it in the air—I knew he was up to no good."

It's a great story, Luke thinks, but it was dumb luck, too. Another guy, less nervous, would have taken his mother out along with the clerk, the opportunity to use the gun twice instead of once an incentive, the old lady lingering even a provocation. But for Louise, he was a young punk about to do something unacceptable! Luke wonders just how aware the guy was of his mother, her staunch disapprobation, whether in fact within the tiny store she reduced him to adolescent status, or whether he was only aware of her as a person who could ID him in a police lineup. He'd like to have been there to observe the dynamic, the guy tossing down the magazine with disgust and leaving, the clerk and Louise in ready, ebullient dialogue with each other, the police on the way.

He wanders back to the kitchen and this time pulls open the oven door, the heat rushing at his face. He lifts out the noisy chicken. Behind him, behind the crackling of chicken fat and olive oil, he can hear them laughing, knows, of course, why they like the story of Louise and the 7-Eleven clerk, a feisty old lady prevailing in a world that barely acknowledges she takes up space—and two young women thinking to themselves, Maybe being an old woman will have some high points, too. He does not want to feel sorry for them, but he does.

"My son," he hears his mother begin, "thinks I tsh-tshed the guy, wagged my finger at him and told him to run along home. I didn't say a word; I just thought, Shoot me, you asshole; that kid who works here barely shaves."

The baster pulls up only about a tablespoon of oil, and as it drips skimpily about the chicken, Luke thinks without really wanting to about Sadie, sees a great nest of twigs enveloping her body as scrawny as a baby bird's. No sound, no struggling for food, the tiny cavern of a mouth empty. There's a fund of fat he finds by tipping the pan and peering into the cavity of the chicken. He pulls it into the baster and somehow he feels better as it falls evenly, glistening down the breasts and beneath the splayed wings.

Sadie, he says to himself, quietly, go away, Sadie. And she does. He's good at making her, allowing her time in his mind, allowing her to have his mind's images, and then shuffling them under and away. They always come to him here—so many images—when he's in this house. He quarters red potatoes, tosses them with olive oil and thyme and spreads them out across a cookie sheet for roasting. He'd wanted to cook halibut or sea bass, but Mingis had been at the seafood counter, and so Luke had taken his twice-selected potatoes and moved down into meats and poultry. Their volleys this morning on the tennis court had been desultory at first, the ball traveling slowly, abjectly from corner to corner, from Mingis's baseline to Luke's. Then Luke showed Mingis he could at least serve, and the game quickened, till anyone observing could see Mingis raging against all he could not change in the world, his shots barely civilized drives so viciously calculated down court lines, Luke chose not to call them, either out or in, letting Mingis have game after game, and when Mingis at last sat on the bench, his head swung down between his knees, his terrified, sweating, tear-soaked face shrouded behind the white club towel, Luke had sat down beside him. "I think Stan is going to get better," Luke said. He had not reached out, had not draped an arm over Mingis's shoulder; he had just continued to talk. "Stan is starting to respond—but if I tell you what all I'm heartened by, I'm not sure you'll exactly see why." And then a drink runner had handed a telephone to Mingis and he had taken the call, standing up from the bench, the towel tossed behind him. Luke sees himself sitting alone on the bench as he recalls the scene, recalls watching Mingis walk out onto the court, talking, Luke waiting, packing his rackets, feeding balls down their canisters, waiting as Mingis walked off the court and down toward the clubhouse. They had had no other exchange, and Mingis never looked back. "Luke, the beloved physician, sends you his greetings," Luke quotes to himself. "Colossians 4:14."

Alice stands next to him in the kitchen, peering down into the bowl of cucumbers. He's trimming pieces of chervil fronds onto the cucumbers with a pair of scissors. The scissors make a slicing, icy sound and Luke thinks, bizarrely, that because of the scissors he and Alice cannot hear the chervil falling and tumbling about the cucumbers, that there's a soft bouncing sound just beneath the shearing of the metal which he can't get to with his ear.

"What is that?" she asks.

"Oh ho," he says. "You don't know chervil?"

She leans down and peers into the oven, then straightens her back. "How many patients do you have? Do you have a lot?"

He can see she wants to be serious. "Yes," he says, "I have a lot. Then I consult on many more. At the center. At St. John's. There's significant attention on autism right now, in the mass media, movies, but whether or not it's more common is arguable.

We may be diagnosing it more, but whether it's autism or not, or whether it's just behaviors we associate with it, I'm not sure —I'm not convinced it's more prevalent . . . though reports are saying that. I think we're better at seeing it earlier, knowing it for what it is earlier, and that's good. But we're also using the term *autism*, when in fact we mean mentally deficit—somehow parents don't mind the term *autism* as much as they do *mentally retarded*. Go figure."

"Do you believe it could be caused by vaccinations?" she asks.

"It's not the vaccination; it's the preservative in the vaccination—thimerosal," Luke replies. "Exposure to mercury, environmental exposure to chemicals—older studies couldn't isolate a particular chemical, but organic mercury compounds seem to be emerging in more recent studies. Mercury pollution. I'd like to know," he says, "but it's not necessarily going to help me treat patients. We know better than to put so many things into the environment, and yet we just go on doing it. Ethyl mercury's in flu shots, too, by the way."

"What's the connection with your sister?" she asks.

The bluntness of the question startles him less than the time she's chosen to ask it—even less than the artlessness of the question's phrasing. He stops scissoring. He moves his weight from one leg to the other. He puts the scissors down on the tile counter, listens to the small clatter they make. A pepper grinder stands near him and so he picks it up and grinds pepper into the cucumbers, enough energy in his elbow to dig postholes. He can't bring himself to say anything; he is afraid his words, the words he wants to speak at this moment, will irreparably damage any chance he has with her. He doesn't understand her callousness, the idea that he could answer such a question kibitzing in the kitchen. He calls forth the physician, switches so consciously, adroitly, it unnerves even in himself a sense of his own honesty. "There is no direct connection," he says coolly, though not coldly, which is how his answer would have sounded had he not toggled himself over into doctor. "Sadie's problems were not within my field—"

"Janey suggested they were," Alice says, interrupting. "That's the last time I depend on her for information."

"And were you—depending on Janey?" he asks.

"Yes, of course," she replies.

He turns to her, standing his full height. "Why?" he questions her, knowing he is letting himself show, letting himself become Luke. "I have a telephone number—obviously, you knew I wanted to see you." The chicken sizzles above the bass of his words; the look on her face is uncomfortable and becoming more so, her eyes dimming; he is fucking up. "It's a beautiful blouse," he says nervously, daffily, then adds, "on you. I like it."

"When my brother and his wife argue, she stands on a chair," Alice says. "So they're the same height."

He pulls a towel off the counter and wipes his hands, then tosses it back without looking. Why don't we just go to bed, he thinks to himself; that evens up the height issue. "You have a brother?" he asks, and then doesn't wait for an answer but says rapidly, "Doesn't she feel absurd standing on a chair, as though she's shrieking about mice?" He's serious, a little angry, but the look that grows across Alice's face is pure amusement.

"You're right," she agrees, "that *is* absurd," but he realizes she's revealed something. They have, in the two times they've met, always been standing. She's sharply aware of being so much shorter than he, a foot, he figures. In his memory, he's never stood over her, never purposefully used it, though he likes looking down across the precise plane of her nose, likes the way her eyelashes rest against her cheeks, each lash particulate and fine as a crack in china. He's six four and knows the gamut of reactions people can have to imposing height. He hunkers down a lot with his patients, though that's because he wants to encourage eye contact, wants to present his face to them—to be *in* their face, as it were. He realizes she usually stands away from him, took her Scotch earlier and walked out into the garden, turned and looked across at him, eye level; she sets a distance between them; she'd also come and stood beside him and looked down into the bowl of cucumbers, the straight dark hair sliding across her cheeks and then swinging back as she turned and looked up at him.

"I played a horrible game of tennis today," he says, and walks across the kitchen to get a different pepper mill, one with a finer grind. "The father of one of my patients—at his club. Sometimes I want to see if I can't glean genetic components to behavior that in the parents somehow got socialized or channeled in such a way as to become passable, or perhaps was just so much milder. Not that I was doing that on the tennis court, but this guy's son, I see him three days a week, and last week Stan walks straight into a wall. He looks up at mc and says, 'Rejected. Not tactical to move forward in a single line.' He then bursts into laughter. In the movie, there's this group of American soldiers about to go behind enemy lines—"

"What do you mean 'in the movie'?"

Luke stops twisting the pepper mill in his hands. He's talking as though Alice were an intimate already. He starts to explain, stammers a bit because he wasn't really wanting to explain about Stan, but, rather, to discuss Stan's father, the tennis he'd played with him—or rather, the wall he'd provided for him to slam balls against. Sometimes Luke himself needs an ear that just goes where he goes, listens, and leaps however he leaps; Sadie is the only person he can remember who didn't need a road map of transitions, explanations, who could wait to know where the hell they were in a conversation—or not wait, but just be there—and she was two years younger than he was and for the last years of her life on drugs too debilitating for adults to be on, let alone a thin teenage girl.

"It's called 'perseverative scripting'—or rather, my patient presents a form of it."

"Do I understand now?" Alice asks him seriously, and Luke can see she's not in the least snide in that question, and that she actually wants to understand. Any doctor knows how to answer a question without answering it, or to get someone to stop asking questions, to deflect the questions in such a way that it seems like they're answered, a form of professional terrorism all doctors know how to deploy, whether they admit it or not, use it or not. Luke hadn't been meaning not to explain—he was going to—but he also realizes someone else might have just left it at that, perseverative scripting. Sure, Doctor, whatever, just tell me when the kid is going to stop doing it!

"Perseverative scripting. It actually might be better characterized as an ability," Luke says carefully, "though how an ability manifests or is enlisted is more likely the locus of illness. Certain children memorize some set script, a television program, or movies, as is my patient's—" Luke stops himself from saying *fixation*, though that would be the traditional word. He finds Stan's use of *The Lion King* and *The Manchurian Candidate* less *fixated* than intricately reasoned out as response. It's a fixation, yes, but Stan's is in *response* to the world outside himself. Luke finds this different from other cases of perseverative scripting, in which children merely recite over and over and over again whatever it is they have latched onto, a maze of sound, though intelligible, which enthralls them. That is a fixation, he thinks, but Stan is actually responding. "My patient uses only sentences from two movies to speak in."

"I went to school with a lot of girls like that," Alice says.

"No." Luke cuts in quickly, too harshly; he wants to say, Don't be flippant, but instead he says, "Don't be wooed by notions of common behavior that are off by just a few degrees—these children are deficit, neurologically, psychologically. More to the point, they're deeply unhappy. Behavior is gauged upon a spectrum, and our sense of behavior can be decidedly relativistic, but these children aren't neurotypical even if you allow a generous range within our sense of normal."

"I think I believe you, Doctor," Alice says, laughing a bit, and Luke can see that she's willing to calm him, to retreat pretty quickly. "I didn't mean to suggest you were poaching from perfectly happy children in order to have a practice."

"You may put the cards away now. Goodbye, Raymond."

Alice looks up at him, her dark eyes confused. She shifts her weight from one heel to the other.

"You may put the cards away now. Goodbye, Raymond."

"I gather that's a line from one of the movies?" she asks.

"Three months, three appointments a week—the only thing he'll say. Thirty-six appointments—'You may put the cards away now. Goodbye, Raymond'—*thirty-six* appointments."

"How many times do they have to see something before they have it memorized?"

Luke is used to people wanting to understand, asking questions, many truly interested, but the questions themselves spring from the wrong place—or rather, from a place of presumed normality. No autistic kid ever sits down to memorize a book or a movie script—their brains are different, receive differently. Luke thinks a better question might be why, when he and Alice watch *The Manchurian Candidate*, they don't have it in their brains complete? Or perhaps they do, but something blocks the "normal" brain from being able to recall it whole or in all its parts. There are stops in the normal brain, stops that autistic children do not always have, though obviously autistic children have other stops, other areas of seemingly complete disengagement.

Where Luke begins in explaining to yet another set of parents, or even to another woman, is always difficult—and sometimes what the hell is he explaining, when he has not even spent more than three hours with a kid, and every kid different? "That's just it," he says, smirking, "they don't memorize it—it's just *there*—or at least in the case of Stan, the movie is just there, and *The Lion King*, too, just there, poof, *there* entire."

"Instant recall?" Alice asks.

"Even *recall* is an equivocal term," Luke says. "It's not like some mental labor is being performed. With some of them, it's as though something encoded is activated—it's there."

"She was autistic, wasn't she, your sister?"

Luke is happy and unhappy and stunned that Alice seems so set on talking about Sadie. But he needs to talk about Sadie; he knows he does. He would like to take Alice's arm and walk her right out the kitchen door onto the circular drive, across the shifting gravel, and load her into his car, and then where? He does not know, but anywhere, the car particulating them from all else in the world in that moment and in that necessity, his necessity, for sure, *his*, but he is unabashed, indeed so unabashed that he almost reaches out his hand . . . but he is also slowed by his astonishment that she is pushing the subject of Sadie. Luke wonders what sort of mechanism is at work in himself that almost nothing a patient says or does startles him, and yet he treads the outside world appalled, and deeply so. He thinks he's missing a general measure of what constitutes civility now. Not that it's his sense of civility, but what passes as such. He starts to say that perhaps they could have a conversation about Sadie at another time, a time when he is not distracted—those would be the words he would use—but he knows he means a time when he can proctor a much harsher control of himself. What happened in this very kitchen a week ago is not going to happen again; it surprised him, his tears, and he wants no more soppiness. Just be a doctor now, Luke, he thinks; just speak your report, that case halfway around the world, someone else's sister, improperly diagnosed, or maybe not, just your cool, professional appraisal.

"Probably," he says. "Autistic, a rare form perhaps? Or perhaps not autistic. We can talk another time—there will *be* another time, won't there?" he asks quickly. "Another time not tonight?"

He watches her say yes, her face lifting up and smiling her yes combined with her wonder that she is saying yes. He can see it is wonder, that she has surprised herself and that she instantly regrets her answer.

"No date," he says.

"No date. Okay," she says, and there's a huskiness in her voice he's not ever heard before. If he's not being melodramatic, and he may well be being such, she's carefully, very firmly controlling some deep uncomfortableness, even perhaps something that borders on terror. "Yes, good, yes," she says, her smile returning. "No date."

"I'm actually not a particularly threatening guy. Ask Janey—course, that's like asking a family member. She may tell you more truth than you want to hear—like 'He's the most pansy-assed guy you'll ever not want to meet.'"

"I better return to the others. Don't you think I'm being rude?" She speaks briskly, passes before him, her velvet pants swishing as she crosses the tile floor. Luke is nonplussed—if he is using that word correctly for once—but he is learning she's not one for transitions between statements and questions, not a pause, about as much sexual tension as one room can hold and then poop, dawdle, and drool, Christ. What an odd creature, and maybe he doesn't need the intricacy of someone like that in his life, but, rather, some big simple girl who will good-naturedly make him some babies and just as good-naturedly raise them on egg salad sandwiches and oatmeal cookies. Just what sct of wings is she waiting in? That would be the question, now wouldn't it? Luke goads himself: It's not like Big Simple Girl has ever heaved her big simple body his way, *either*, though that is not exactly accurate, and he squirms a bit even now in recalling Betsy, and then Katherine, women from so many years ago now, women he had liked and even loved and never invited to stay, not that he's been a shit, at least not a total shit, but he hurt them both, and hurt them enough to know it was a pretty sorry thing to do, and disturbingly easy when contrarily his vanity runs to more difficult endeavors. But even so, *industrial flowers*, mechanical flowers? And yet he can't help himself, sees that small foot in its small black shoe perched on its chair rung— perched? Maybe perched, but maybe fixed, too, lodged, as insistent on its chair rung as a bee on a lavender stem. He loves her seriousness, her avidity, and yet how easily humorous she is, how confident. He knows he expected some much more gnarled difficulty in her affect, but it just isn't there.

He hears the sounds of their conversation from the garden, Louise and Alice and Janey, the murmurs and swells. He pulls the second oven open and slides the potatoes in on their cookie sheet. He likes their red-skinned backs slicked with oil, but the heat coming from the oven doesn't feel hot enough, and he looks at the gauge. It reads 400. He'll have to ask Louise about the calibration. He wants not to feel as resentful as he does in this moment about Alice's allegiance to the company of Janey and his mother. But just how is she being rude if he is alone slaving away in the kitchen? What miniaturist note of etiquette did he miss this time?

Yet he knows what note it is, knows she doesn't want him moving so fast, maybe doesn't want him moving at all. He's back on her loft floor, seeing the huge moat of empty space surrounding her table. If he can't decipher what those vast reaches of square footage mean, he's no doctor.

He pulls the corks on a couple of bottles of Lynch-Bages. God knows he wasn't drinking what Janey brought—what had she brought anyway? He walks across the kitchen to the bottles standing near the sink. Oh, probably they're quite drinkable, he has to admit, Napa Valley cabs made by a solid though heavy-handed vintner. Janey had advertised swill, but they're far better than that. He wonders what she paid for them, worries that she dropped a whole day's pay on two bottles—Alice couldn't pay her much, could she? At least Janey had eaten well when she'd been here more constantly; at least she'd gone to doctors Luke knew and been taken care of; at least . . . But he does not finish his thought, because Janey is standing there beside him, punching him in the arm affectionately, her face surrounded by hair the colors of plastic fruit, yellow and lime and orange.

"I hope you've made some progress," she whispers in his ear conspiratorially.

"Maybe you could tie her down for me, Janey," Luke says without humor or spirit. "And don't spend your hard-earned money on wine next time. You know you don't have to bring wine to this house, just yourself—and what made you change your mind about me making passes at your boss?"

Janey stands looking at him. Her hazel eye is almost as dark now as the eye he thinks of as graphite. He can tell she wishes she hadn't said anything, and there's an apology on her lips about to be spoken.

"Stop drinking sports drinks," he says quickly. "It's changing your hair color. And God knows you've got confused hair—"

Janey laughs and springs about the kitchen the way Luke is used to, and yet he notices it tonight because it's been awhile since he's been here with Janey as she drapes and straightens and slides and skips, her body never quite still, but not manic, either, and never stiff, just buoyant, brisk, happy. *Happy*, Luke thinks, really happy, and he's never unamazed by this fact: Janey seems genuinely a happy person, and though there were early days in which he kept a close eye out for fissures in the sweetness, a dark psychological key to the constantly changing hair color, he's never found a thing to suggest anything but Janey's seemingly unwavering joy with the world as she knows it now, living with Louise, and even more recently working with Alice Samara.

"Yeah, so why aren't pregnant women supposed to dye their hair?" Janey asks. "I was wondering about that the other day, and I couldn't remember, and I thought, Shit, do I have chemicals coursing through my veins or something, or dye sitting on my brain, But then I thought, They pump people up full of dye in the hospital and watch it go through their bodies, so what's the difference?"

"Oh, no difference, of course, they're pushing Clairol down at Cedars-Sinai, no question about it."

"Yeah, yeah," Janey says, "never a straight answer from the mama's boy."

"Barium sulfate, you want a straight answer, which shows up on X rays— So where does she live?" Luke asks. "Have you ever been there?"

"What do you mean, have I ever been there? *You've* been there, you doofus."

Luke pulls tongs from a crock of utensils by the stove and draws open an oven door. Janey hands him a hotpad. "Thanks," he says absently. "That area has residential zoning?" he then asks. "How can that be?"

"Did you come down the birth canal with a tie on or something! Residential zoning? Stay on task, Luke. Let's talk about Alice, not city code."

Luke ignores Janey's sarcasm. "She has a brother," he states, turning the potato quarters, exposing their pale sides. "I found that out."

"Even I didn't know that."

"So, where do I take her? Not a date—tell me where we should go. She'll see me, but not a date."

"I have the feeling *she'll* take you," Janey says, winking her hazel eye at him. "Put these in the dining room?" she asks, holding up the two bottles of wine Luke has opened. Luke nods, and for the rest of the evening he nods, barely speaking, barely called upon to speak, outnumbered, he supposes, though what seems most operative is a keen lack of interest in anything he might say. He concedes that there is a little more interest in what he *does*, as it is Luke who is carving the chicken and pushing potatoes off the cookie sheet into a bowl, Luke who is filling wineglasses, Luke who is mashing roasted garlic into a small dish with olive oil and salt. But after this, after the preparations and the serving, conversation quickly drifts to eddy about the three of them, and Luke listens and is quiet.

Sadie has been dead twenty-one years this March, he thinks, as every year he thinks this sentence, and thinks it many many times throughout the month, only the number changing; Sadie has been dead two years this March; Sadie has been dead five years this March. Then it seemed that through medical school, he did not think it so much, did not mount the tabulation, but then the sentence started up again at the institute and during his second residency, occurred to him more regularly than it had for years: Sadie has been dead ten years this March; Sadie has been dead eleven years this March, dead of acute peritonitis that seemed only to make her right leg move oddly, the alchemical power of the autistic mind to transubstantiate pain. Anybody else would have been screaming maniacally for days, but she appeared *happy* that last night, laughing with Luke over her new jig, speeding it up, her face in full flush. Would he have tumbled to it had he entered her bedroom and stood over her bed? Would he have felt her body burning up with fever? He might have, he answers the ubiquitous inquest, certainly he might have, but he didn't like going into Sadie's bedroom with its massively confrontational artwork, the yards and yards of butcher paper extending up across the ceiling and down the other wall, the huge looming figures outlined along the paper edges and singling you out as you came into the room. After Sadie died, it took four months for him to finally push open the door and find the room closed in upon itself like a blown magnolia, the huge lengths of paper having pulled from the ceiling—four months for him to step into the room and close the door and sit down within the folds and volutes and look closely for the first time at the intricately conceived maps and the complicated diagrams filling the arms and legs and stomach cavities of the huge figures.

He is aware now as he drinks his wine in the dining room that Sadie's room is just above his head, and though the maps and diagrams are no longer there, his visit to her room that day will always be for Luke the specific point in time and space when he decided he would do what he does, and decided further that no production of anyone's mind would ever scare him again, that no art could ever be as dangerous as the mind that denies looking at it, denies attempting to read it and understand it. He hadn't cried sitting within the massive volutions of white paper covered with Sadie's mind. He cries now, he thinks, but he hadn't cried then, sixteen, tall and good-looking, bright, "the laziest child God ever let live," and proud of it every time his mother said it, and then she never said it again, did not have to, too lazy to cry for his own sister, too lazy to penetrate the strangeness of her room to stand above her bed in the volcanic heat coming off her body, too lazy to get her to a hospital. These are all constructions of his mind, he knows—knows that Louise never thought those things.

"She doesn't seem a little removed to you?" his mother had asked him. "She doesn't seem—I don't know, but don't her cheeks seem pinker, fuller?" And he'd said, "It's the drugs, Mom, and anyway, how could she be any more removed than she is?" Luke was sixteen, cooler than cool, instructing his mother in the secondary effects of the various drugs Sadie was on. He and his buddies had gotten their hands on every bit of literature they could find, gleefully presenting their social studies project on the outrageous arbitrariness of legalized versus criminalized drugs. They knew more about the adverse effects of antipsychotics than they did about the girls seated next to them in their classes. In fact, Luke was the one to tell his mother that Sadie's positive pregnancy test was probably inaccurate, and not just because he knew that Sadie had never had a sexual relation with anyone in her *entire* life but also because Prolixin could occasionally cause a false positive. So he had credibility with his mother, more than a little during the days when Sadie was dying from a ruptured appendix that no one knew she had, least of all Sadie, who kept pulling her leg up in a new funny hitched jig that Luke had never seen Sadie do before, but which amused them both.

Today, if he saw that pulling movement of the leg in a patient, in any child, he'd know there was something awry in the peritoneal cavity, and he'd know to trust his instincts, a mother's instincts—so what if the child didn't respond to palpation, so what! At sixteen, he learned the extent to which autistic withdrawal could expunge cathexis not only of the external world but the internal world, as well. But he could not have known, perhaps no one could have known, that the fifteen hours she slept that night and into the generally sleepy Sunday afternoon were not the protracted hours of teenage slumber lengthened even further by prescribed drugs, but, rather, a deepening coma, the peritonitis raging completely untreated because Sadie had never suggested to anyone that she was uncomfortable, let alone in pain. She'd said good night, doing her silliness with her leg, and kind of goofily distracted "Hey? Luka Bazooka, When pigs fly! Pie in the sky! In a pig's eye!" the leg pulling up, the leg pulling up, the leg pulling up. He can see it before him as clearly as he can see the dark pendulum of Alice's hair across her shoulders.

Luke had cried last week in this house's kitchen. He'd cried for himself; he understands that. He will not deny melodrama or vanity, will not even try to make it other than it is. He feels he's paid, done his time of guilt, even meted out some blame, it would seem, and unwisely. Now he'd like to stop all that, and to stop paying, too; he's not even chagrined by this crass terminology. He stares down the dining room table at Alice. Her face is animate; she is talking, but he does not hear. Her small fingers rest against her wineglass, and the other hand—he is sure of it—rests in her lap, the thumb tucked snugly into its fist. She's thirty what? he wonders. Janey's twenty-three going on twelve, his mother's seventy, he's thirty-seven, and, the Lynch-Bages is '90. Maybe she's thirty-four or thirty-five; he can't tell, nor does it particularly matter to him, but he still ventures a few guesses, and later, when he walks her to her car beneath the dense gloom of the ficus trees, he wonders again, pulling her age down to thirty-one or thirty-two, a comment about liking to jog at night, which strikes him as youthful foolishness, and then the car, which even in the darkness looks to be bright orange—lipstick orange—a kid's jalopy L.A.–style, a Ford Falcon, but *cherry*. "Tell me, please tell me, you've got a car phone," he says.

"I do," she says simply. Then she half laughs and half gulps. "And a gun. I have that, too."

Luke could've done without hearing the last. "May you never be called upon to use it," he says. He knows he sounds like an old fart, but guns are not something he has much love of, having done a psychiatric residency with the son of one of Wyoming's biggest ranchers, a brilliant clinician and rich and given to games of Russian roulette after telephone conversations with his mother. Luke was sure he was fucking her—had been since he was a teenager.

"Maybe you should live in a better neighborhood," he says. "Actually just starting with a neighborhood would help."

"More people live down there than you think."

Luke watches her put the key in the door's lock and turn it. He wants her hand to fidget so she can't fit the key, but it's not nerves that animate Alice; it's speed, quickness, a sureness of movement Luke keeps nudging into neurosis. He'd described Alice's hands to his mother as "nervous," but he thinks now that that is an inaccuracy on his part, a wish for a fragility that is not there. She's certainly had a past, and certainly the strangeness of her flowers stems from some crinkle somewhere, some trauma, but she is not in need of any psychiatrist's couch; he can see that. And the absence of this need perplexes him a bit, leaves him stripped of his usual . . . advantages, he admits.

He doesn't want her to leave. He glances behind and sees Janey's face in the kitchen window above the sink. She is talking to Louise, seemingly not paying any attention to what is beyond in the drive. It's rather spectacular how like a parrot's plumage her hair appears in the bright rectangle of the window.

"You resent me having Janey, don't you?" Alice says abruptly.

She's caught him looking back, and she's read the glance all wrong, though maybe her words are correct. He just doesn't particularly want Janey and his mother doing the gawk at the window, not that he was going to pin Alice against the car and put his tongue down her throat. "No," he says, "no, you're wrong. My mother and I are very pleased that Janey works for you, and she seems to like it very much. If there's any resentment, it's Janey's resentment against people taking up your time. Janey's very protective of you—it took me months to get those directions—and then she was incensed I'd asked you out. It doesn't seem to me like you need much protection, so how about tomorrow? It's Sunday. But you come to me," he says. "I'm not going through that gauntlet again."

"Yes," she says without question or hesitation. Yes, sitting down in her car, he is in charge, and then she is there the next morning in his doorway, holding a long funnel of brown paper from which emerges sprays of bell-shaped orange flowers he has never seen before. Even the color is an unfamiliar shade.

"*Sandersonia*," she says in answer to the question on his face.

"Ah," he says.

"Australian." And this time he does not intone anything, but, rather, steps aside and watches her enter his house, her face reflected for an instant in the hall mirror, and it means something huge to him and he thinks it very likely, in the next few moments, that he will make a complete fool of himself. But then she doesn't seem to be watching him right now, and he relaxes a bit and starts toward the kitchen for something to put the flowers in, but she produces from a string bag he's not seen hanging down her back a tall reed of green bamboo, which just happens to hold water.

"Oh," he manages to say, "yeah, thank you," and they are now in the kitchen and she's pouring a river of black stones into the bamboo for ballast. Where on her person were those black stones? Luke wonders. She moves to the sink and he reaches across to pull on the water after she has put the length of bamboo beneath the faucet. He likes her in his kitchen, wants already to say, You look good in this house, but he knows he can't say anything so rash, so obvious. "Enough?" he asks, and she murmurs yes and he pushes the water off.

"Hi, Luke," she says, looking up at him, smiling, *hi* because he's looking at her with inquiry on his face. Or perhaps evaluation? *Hi* to say, Yes, so what do you see? He laughs, and then she says, "I like that, how easily you laugh, at yourself. It's not very doctorly, Doctor."

"Really?" he says, and he watches her shake her head, the straight dark hair twirling gently around her face.

"Maybe one can be smug about gallbladders," he ventures, "but not what I do." He doesn't really think about doctors that much, what they are or should be, how they act in the world. At least he doesn't think he does. He supposes he used to, maybe. When he was being shrunk, he used to think about sanity. At Columbia during the psych residency, he used to think he'd never met a psychiatrist he thought fit to take over the care of anyone else's mental health. "I spent years working rather hard not to think about what it was to be a psychiatrist," he says to Alice; "I mean what it meant personality wise. One of my fellow residents played Russian roulette on a regular basis; another had her teeth pulled out because she thought their roots were growing up into her skull—and both were brilliant psychiatrists."

"Isn't that accurate, though, about the roots growing into the skull?" she asks.

"Accurate if you don't think they're trying to strangle your brain."

"Oh," she says, raising her dark eyebrows. Luke watches her cut the ends off the flowers with shears, which she has also produced from somewhere.

"Yes, *oh*. I've never forgotten her. Denise Asnes, about as gluttonous with food as she was with books. I once actually watched her try to take a bite out of a book—the sandwich was in her other hand. She had all these books spread about her—she was reading several at once—but the one she was focused on was lying on the table and she held another in her hand. There she was trying to tear away at *Autistic States in Children*. I can still see her teeth bearing down on the tall black letters of Frances Tustin's name."

"I guess doctors do have weird stories," she says, and he is pleased that she remembers their exchange how many months ago now.

He's had whitefish and smoked salmon delivered from Factor's Delicatessen, bagels, cream cheese. He's run to the store for capers, a red onion, tomatoes, mineral water. His garden is a mess, but he's got a table back there and chairs, and though he's never managed cushions for their fiercely uncomfortable iron seats, he hasn't dragged the pillows from his bed to pad them, either. It doesn't matter that the table and chairs are good, French, a gift from Louise—pillows from his bed in rumpled pillowcases would make them look shabby. He doesn't want that look of bachelor habitats, which is always a bit too close to the look of a boys' fort, furniture too happily scavenged from an alley, too happily made to work, and a barrenness next to some unabashed hoard, a lone jar of mustard in the refrigerator but two shelves bulging with microwave popcorn. He just doesn't want to appear provisional.

"It's a sweet house," Alice says as she moves the tall stems around in the bamboo vase, and Luke supposes it is, but it's also the house he was compelled to buy and he can't ever quite leave that be. Louise and Janey live alone in 4,500 square feet, but Luke would obviously be cooking women in acid were he to live there with them! *You live with your mother*—the horror on women's faces, though they would be simultaneously saying, "How nice. What a comfort that must be to her. With a house like that, why not?" Luke can't decide whether to be more disgusted with the culture or with himself for complaining, when *indeed* he had the means to buy a house in Los Angeles in the first place. White man blues, boo hoo, but he has not had time for a house, and certainly not a yard or a garden, and he hates that Alice will look at this and think it's how he wants to live, a physicalization of his psyche. Finally he says, and far too long after Alice has spoken, "Yes, it could be a sweet house, but I don't have time—you'll be appalled by the garden."

"I'm not a good gardener myself," she says, laughing. "I let others do that work."

Luke realizes he's assumed Louise's talents are Alice's and he's abashed, if not a bit disturbed. She ain't your mother, he tells himself. Still, he thinks, Alice will be as unhappy as Janey and his mother were at the dead plumerias, both plants probably forty years old and now dead from Luke's neglect. Louise had looked with complete wonder: "They don't even *like* a lot of water!"

"I ordered some lox and bagels from the deli," Luke says. "I hope that appeals—some whitefish, too." He pulls a platter from the refrigerator, starts to gather plates and silverware.

"Could I see the rest of the house first?" she asks him, and he stops abruptly, his hands hovering over the silverware drawer. This woman makes him nervous and he does not like it, but there is also something new in this nervousness that excites him—that even reignites some interest he might have had in the past in himself.

"Not much to see," he says, but of course he's straightened the place up like a maniac this morning, using an entire roll of paper towels for the bathroom—what does the maid do?—and heaving boxes of patient files into the garage, where he has meant to put them for months now. He thought to change the sheets on the bed but then hooted himself into sensibility; hope springs delusional. He had looked into his den and thought *no way*, then pulled the door shut, but of course it's the door Alice grows interested in after the living room and dining room and breakfast room.

"Den," he says. "A real mess."

"The room you like best?" she asks, but she is actually noting this, and it *is* the room he likes best, this is true. He is curious to see if she urges to see it, but instead she reaches out and swings the door open herself and peers in. "Now this is interesting," she says, and Luke has to laugh. He smells her perfume, sandalwood, he thinks, and something else; he is no expert on scent, but it appeals to him, this deep richness—it mollifies him, even.

"Do your patients ever come here?" she asks.

Only you come here, Luke thinks to himself, an odd, seemingly senseless thought. It's been a little while since anyone but Louise, and occasionally Janey, has been here—but not in this room. No one but Luke comes in here. The maid comes to the house, her thin blond hair hanging down in her face, the mother of four who cleans for a living, she comes, Mondays and Fridays, but after that, the entire place is solely visited by Luke. *Visited,* he thinks, the right word. "No," he says aloud, "in this day and age, that would probably be folly, particularly if something were to happen, and with autistic kids—and all stripes of autistic kids—there's a lot of clumsiness and, because of it, injury, minor usually, but nonetheless, you wouldn't want to be called into suspicion. Stan, the little boy I was telling you about last night. The other day, he's standing right in front of a door that is sooner or later going to swing open and knock him pretty hard. Today, black eyes, we don't think *what*; we think *WHO*."

"But parents must know they have kids who are particularly prone—"

She can't be that naïve, can she? Luke wonders, but then he *does* know far more about what parents seize upon than most. "It may have something to do with the history of the treatment of autism, too," he says. "There was a lot of restraint in the first therapies, behavior modification, but it appears brutal to us now, even, ironically, as we return to some forms of restraint. But bruises, black eyes, scratches—believe me, we live in inquisitional times, and I already seem too unorthodox to some."

"I believe you, Doctor," she says, turning back to him, smiling. "I really like this room. You should put the *Sandersonia* in here."

"Okay, I will," he says, and he's happy as he says it, and calm. "I will," and he wonders what she sees here among the hundreds of books and files, the two computers, the old institutional desk, as ugly an oak as any ever hewn, and orange, with a grain like oiled feathers.

"I'll get them," she says, brushing past him in the doorway, and when she returns, the thin green stems flounce in the breeze she makes in her briskness. "Here?" she asks, moving toward the desk, but the small orange bells are already there, waving up and down, settled into the desk's only canyon of uncovered surface. "I brought them for you, so I thought they should be placed where you actually *are*," she says, looking up at him, and he sees that she says this apologetically because she feels she's invaded, infiltrated too far a personal territory into which she wasn't invited.

"Don't worry about it," he says. "It's fine." And then, perhaps ill-advisedly, he goes on. "My sense of you is that the last place in the world that would interest you is a space someone constructed for others to see. You're interested in private space, forts, hideaways, the backs of closets, maybe the forest—or lairs within it."

"You do this a lot?" she asks, moving past him again. This time, her passage is different, less swift, less assured. Why what he has said has made her feel bad, he doesn't understand.

As Luke pulls the door shut, he sees Stan drawing wildly in the air above the desk, and he sees the orange *Sandersonia* bells working carefully a detail into the corner of that air. "Yeah," he says to her, "I do this a lot—it's what I do," and he imagines Polly Markens standing there beside Alice, Polly's face beneath the brooding eaves of blond curls, Polly's body as taut as a scream, but her face—once he can sort it from the hair—her face is turned up to Alice, watching avidly as the rope of sweet peas grows longer and denser: a mantle . . . and then what protects Polly is some densely bowered surround bigger than she is, greater, and Polly is unafraid and whole within it, her body distinct from what protects it, and Polly understanding, knowing where her body ends and the mantle begins . . . .

Alice and he sit in the garden, such as it is, and eat and Alice asks for a hat, which he brings her, a cap really, from a winery up north where he's bought many a case of wine. She looks funny in it and he wants her to take it off, misses the gleam of her hair in the easy spring sunlight, actually rushes them a bit through lunch in order to get her out of the sun and out of this dumb hat. They drive up the coast, and Luke tries to answer her questions, which come unadorned, without finesse, their bluntness softened only by what seems her true interest in the answers. He wants to pose his own questions, about *eighty* of them at this point, but she's elusive down to her last chromosome, and so he lets her run ahead of them both, her habit of statement and then, without pause, question. "And so after Sadie died, which must have been horrible, where did your father go?" And he relays to her as best he can the gradualism of those days, the emotional diminution that attacked them all, though slowly, almost quietly, until his parents had no responses left for each other, neither affectionate nor bitter, but only a flatline of speechlessness.

"I remember my father leaving across the gravel of the drive," he tells her. "Seven crunches before he reached his car door—"

"You counted?" she asks.

"Yes, I counted, and I've remembered that number all these years, as though I were a little boy watching helplessly—but of course I wasn't that little. And I've tried to hear that sound of his shoes on the gravel as bitter, or hopeful, anything, any emotion, but it always remained the sound of my parents' numbness, my own even, I guess."

He doesn't tell her how the numbness persisted through his last years of high school, how he fucked anything he could find, and shot heroin and loved the heroin and its pristine needle so much that ironically it presented the one thing that saved him, that alarmed him enough to demand of himself a response. He hadn't been raised to moralize against people who took themselves out of pain, and yet he was confused in those years by so much. Now, he does tell Alice about how he hated the drugs they'd given Sadie, their ability to gut her head, to make her compliant.

"She stopped resembling any aspect of Sadie that I recognized—she didn't entertain herself with her merciless critiques, her barrages, her harangues. Perhaps she wasn't in pain any longer, either. Perhaps she was happier medicated, but I hated that spongy calm—and she would have hated it, too. If she'd been herself." He almost reaches out and pounds the steering wheel. "I didn't know what to hate, or whom to hate, but I began to feel there was something principled in outrage, in Sadie's outrage, and that there was something wrong when we turned our backs on it, pathologized it."

He doesn't say—because he doesn't know how to explain—that cold-blooded sanity, the kind all around us all the time, scared him much more than outrage.

The blue-green haze of sunlight facets the water, and his car moves them sleekly up the coast, and there is no room within this bright light now to tell Alice about the heroin, about the girls, about the outrage which became his, which he took to owning. He tells her more fully about his father leaving, and then his father missing and never heard from again; he tells her about leaving himself for college and then medical school and then one residency after another, and research. Sure he was a good student, an up and coming doctor, and yes, what he does now, in private practice, is not standard, is backed up by only a few decades of study and perhaps promises little, but he says—struggles to say—struggles as carefully as he can to say, that no therapeutic response, psychodynamic or behavioralist, generalized beyond a particular patient in a particular moment of that patient's construction *could* ever be—in his evaluation—very successful for any other patient. "But that also makes me a crackpot in a lot of people's eyes," he adds somewhat sadly. "I think the motivation of the research in a field like autism is problematic. The research assumes from its inception that somewhere either physiologically or neurologically there is a source of disorder, which can then be assumed as the source of disorder in an entire population of patients. The more we push for it, the more we say, 'Oh it is this,' 'Oh it is that,' the stupider we become about the disorder and how it manifests individually."

"I think I believe you, Doctor," she says, and he looks across at her in the seat where just a week ago Louise had sat.

She looks bigger sitting there than she does standing, and the absurd hat is gone. Luke's happy to be driving. Bolting from L.A. was smart—her hands are still, the thumbs tucked up within their fists.

"We spent a number of years changing every kid's brain chemistry," he continues, "only to find it helps some and submerges others even deeper. Couldn't we all have predicted that? It's too intricate a fortress to bring down with just chemistry. We all fight our chemistry differently."

"*Fortress,*" she repeats, "that's an interesting term—"

"It's not mine," he says too sharply.

"All right," she says, and then the car is quiet for a time, and Luke is uncomfortable, more so than it appears she is, and he thinks to remedy something from last night, not so much to set it straight as to explain why it can't be set straight.

"Last night, I said my sister's problems weren't in my field—that's true, and it probably isn't true, too. I don't think we'll ever really have a way of knowing, but first you should understand that many autistic children are not all that intelligent, not the ones I work with privately, but many. Sadie's IQ was fairly high, I'd guess. I've actually never known, which doesn't mean she wasn't autistic, but her behavior argues against autism. She was quite outwardly turned, which is not so of autistic children as a rule. I'd have to say she was ferociously responding to the external world. On the other hand, what Sadie really died from would have caused excruciating pain in someone without severely . . . ." Luke pauses, searching for a term not so scientific, a term to replace *severely inadequate peripheral pain sensitivity*. "Withdrawn" is what he finally says, "in someone not so seriously withdrawn."

"What about hormones?" Alice asks. "Wasn't she fourteen?"

It's a good question and Luke likes it that she's come up with it. Hormone imbalances have always been a real consideration for Luke, but hormone research was not in the dark ages then. It would have been one of the first things the doctors checked— though there's nothing about it in her files—and anyway, Sadie was Sadie as a toddler, long before adolescence, her menarche.

"What do you know about that?" Luke asks her. "It's a good question," but before she responds, before she says, "I don't know anything about it," before she says, "I only know sometimes in some women, some girls, there's more craziness than in others, or a type of craziness," before she hedges and stammers and says, "I don't mean to use the word *crazy*, but hysteria," before all these words are finished coming from her mouth, Luke relives the most horrible memory he has of Sadie, her terror at her body emptying out of her. He'd heard commotion above and bounded the stairs three at a time, but the door to her bedroom was closed, and when he tried it gently, it was locked. He heard his mother with Sadie, soothing her, but Sadie was screaming furiously, horrifically. He doesn't want to knock, doesn't want to be in this house. He hates his sister, hates that he's locked out of her room and can't be inside it with her, hates the muffled sounds of his mother's soothing. He wants her to succeed, to have Sadie quieted within her arms, but Sadie will not allow anyone's arms, and she screams so long, he knows they will have to sedate her, knows he has to call her doctors, perhaps even an ambulance, all the apparatus and personnel that have never helped his sister before, and he slides down the wall and struggles to his feet, all in one motion. He waits through a battery of secretaries, then nurses, and finally a doctor is on the line asking Luke to explain to him what is wrong, but Luke can't exactly do that, as he's not been inside Sadie's bedroom, he has only the screaming to describe, its duration, its pitch. "You have no idea what has caused this?" the doctor asks him impatiently, and Luke says no, no he does not. He's calling because his sister has been screaming for seventeen minutes without stop. He's not calling to inform the doctor of his, Luke's, diagnosis—he is fifteen fuckingyearsold!

Now, in the sedative quiet of the car, he says, "Hormones could have been contributive at a later point, certainly. But maybe what she was was psychotic. She was treated for it, medicated for it, a horrible drug, one never used for children, but somehow used for her. God knows."

Maybe she was both, Luke thinks to himself. No rules in this game ever say you can't have a ruptured appendix because you have an aberrant brain. That was the beautiful irony, wasn't it, Luke thinks, appendix. You're sure you're reading a book about autism, but right when you think you have diagnostic resolution, SURPRISE, a little entry—an appendix—at the back of the book: peritonitis due to infection caused by a ruptured appendix—no shit, and you thought you had this thing licked just by sticking to the chapters on autism.

"Do you see it all around you?" she asks. She twists beneath her seat belt, so that she's sitting almost sideways, looking directly at him, and the belt stretches taut over her far shoulder. Luke likes how she looms in his peripheral vision, how already she's willing him to talk, willing him to terra firma beyond his mind. He likes how she doesn't sit back in chairs, not even against the car seat for very long. He likes the rapt, sentient agility of her body, wonders how she looks asleep.

"Autism?" He looks over again to see if that is what she means. "Do I see autism all around me? No," he says to her nodding head, "no, but it's tempting at times. The ad nauseum of individualism is a type of . . ." and Luke looks for a word, or a phrase. "Mindlessness of others," he says, "but finally that's not like autism. It would be a highly fanciful analogy, even if I've made it myself a couple of times."

"But don't you—" she begins to ask, and he interrupts her.

"I'm sorry—but depending on intelligence, autistic people can be painfully aware that they're not normal—what we call "normal"—but they have a very hard time understanding why they're not normal. You have to explain to them why their conduct seems bizarre to other people, or impolite or rude. There's no conscious decision to behave in antisocial ways because autistics don't start with a concept of what constitutes bad behavior."

"Other children do?" she asks.

"Sure," he says. "They're responsive pretty much instantly to what others think."

"But they're not born with it?"

"Probably they are, or at least born with the brain a certain way—responsive in a certain way. Normal children gain more and more social awareness as they develop. This isn't necessarily true of autistics, or it can take them much, much longer. One of the huge problems with intelligent autistics is how others perceive their behavior, how we in the general population label it. We'll say quite readily, "That's malicious behavior," or we call it "sadistic," or "belligerent," but those words strongly suggest the person being "malicious" understands the feelings of others—or has a consciousness of how to influence others. This awareness just doesn't seem to be what able autistics are capable of."

Out of the corner of his eye, he watches her settle back down against her seat. He thinks she's about to get to something she's wanted to for some time now. "That day you came to the studio," she begins, and her voice is severe, flinty, "you said something about atavism and people hiding in the vegetation after the bombs in Japan and you seemed to liken it to something in the flowers that I do."

Luke realizes—though how he could have missed it is astonishing—that Alice had not exactly loved his comment, that in the moment in her studio, she had said she found it interesting, but that upon reflection, several months' worth, she has not been at all happy with it, with him. Still, Luke is perplexed. If he sees asylum in her work rather than the usual show of beauty, what's to be spurned about that? He's not suggesting pathology. Or violence . . . though of course he is, he chides himself. Some experience or event is back there, distant in her past perhaps, but there, and it hugely influences her work.

He looks over at her hands, the thumbs tucked into her fists. Hadn't she claimed this was genetic? He looks back to the road, to the expanse of lanes and only here and there a car. What he meant by telling her the detail about Hiroshima was really an inquiry, a question to her. What he's seen in her designs is asylum, almost a desperation for it, and he wonders why. But he lets it go, retracts the analogy, "The Japanese, their gardening, perhaps it was just something they knew, a deeply consoling construct of their culture, or perhaps it was atavistic. I've always been interested in the phenomenon, if it can be called that, but it doesn't apply to you, I can see."

She doesn't make any response to him and her face is turned toward her window. "I don't know exactly what does apply to you," he says, fishing. He knows one thing, that she has a brother, and beyond that, very little actual detail. "Parents," he finally says, "where are they?"

"I don't think you'll be meeting them anytime soon." Her voice sounds flat, even tired.

"Okay," he says. "That's fine."

"It's not you, Luke. Jesus, you're sort of infinitely presentable."

"Okay," he says again

They drive as far as Ventura, then Carpinteria. "You need gas," she says, and after he pulls off near Santa Barbara and fills the gas tank, he waits for her to come back from the rest room and watches a scrawny-hipped dog run between the pumps, approaching several people quizzically and then bounding to the door of the men's rest room as it opens. But the dog is not looking for this person, either, this man with his wet suit half stripped off, the rubber arms flailing about his thighs, and Luke wonders where the dog's owner is and remembers the day he first went to see Alice. There was a dog at that gas station, too, on Alameda, alone and nervous, leaping about between the pumps. Probably that dog had been looking for his owner also, but Luke had not noted this then, had himself been too much in search of something that morning to fathom the dog's behavior. All the dog world is asunder, he thinks. Will the dogs ever find their owners, or each other? He doesn't know of anyone who has dogs who are a couple, a male and a female, mates. He feels a momentary heaviness in his chest, some absurd shadowy sadness he didn't know he harbored for dogs.

When Alice emerges from the rest room, he watches her cross the concrete. It's as though her footfalls are fingers making their way up his legs. He can feel her within his thighs. She wears almost exactly what she wore the day he first saw her: a white shirt, black pants, low heels. It must be her "uniform." The dog runs to her and prances around her legs. He wags his long brown tail and leaps in the air, and when she bends to pet him, he bounds off, a furtive glance backward as he charges across the lot. A car starts to pull out and the dog shrinks swiftly out of its way, and then the dog is gone behind a Dumpster and down the alley.

"Cowboy dog," she says, laughing, and Luke wonders how two people observing the precise same thing can have such divergent reactions. The dog has made Luke worry. He imagines the speeding car, witless and brutal as it strikes, the whimpers, the dog's eyes struggling with what has happened. He opens the door for her, watches her sit down and then lift her legs in the way women do, held together as if one fin, like a mermaid. Even wearing pants, she gets in a car this way. Valets must have some stories, though, he thinks. The bird's-eye view.

How far they should drive occupies Luke's thoughts as he turns the key in the ignition. He's surprised his beeper is quiet, and he's grateful. He likes this time with her, wants an expanse of days available to them, some broad somber beach of time within which they might perform all the choreography of courtship. He thinks his way up a map of the coast, Goleta, Isla Vista, Refugio, Gaviota. Isn't there one more state beach? He can't come up with it. Refugio, yes, then there's Gaviota, but there's another in there somewhere, closer, one he's smoked a lot of dope on. It's late afternoon and the sun is in his eyes and he thinks starting back down the coast will be good.

"Ninety-three million miles away and it's still in my eyes," he says.

"You better hope it is," she quips, and he likes that answer, its lilt, its poke. El Capitán comes to him, the beach after Isla Vista. He asks her if she'd like to stop, stretch her legs, walk on a beach. "El Capitán will come up soon, but depending on how far we want to go, there's Refugio, then Gaviota; after that, we should turn back." She shoots a look at him and he knows what she's thinking, that he seems to know the beaches particularly well. He starts to tell her about being a teenager, hanging out at the ocean, boastfully inventive bongs, reading philosophy, *Being and Time*, but instead he says, "Autistic people have a special relationship to water. It can run the gamut from terror to solace; nonetheless, it's often striking. I've been to all these beaches because of Sadie—and many, many times. She loved the ocean, the air, the sound of the waves. Something about the vastness of that sound."

After awhile, he says, "Really, most autistic children are comforted by the sea, by swimming, not frightened of it. Several of my patients draw underwater pictures—though some have creatures in them, threatening ones."

Green-and-white highway signs for Goleta, Isla Vista, the University of California whisk past. Luke eyes the fuel gauge. He likes the tank so full they could drive as far as Carmel, Monterey, Santa Cruz. They can have all the geography a tank of gas will allow them, and even the thought of this provides a terrain, makes him happy, relaxes him.

"Sadie once had a very bad tantrum on a beach," he says. "Someone had a radio. I was embarrassed and my mother and I just had to get her out of there. The radio was on very low; in fact, I couldn't really hear it, but she could—she was such an amazing listener. That may strike you as a funny equation to make," he adds quickly, "that just because she was sensitive to sound—hypersensitive—she was a listener, but she was. Did you know that Schopenhauer thought there was a link between intelligence and sensitivity to sound, which would mean that as a culture, we're raving idiots!"

"Schop—who, Doctor?" She laughs, then says, "No, I do know who you mean, but I've never read him."

"Doesn't matter. He was a philosopher anyway, not a scientist, and yet I've always been struck by that idea. It's total hogwash, and yet somehow it's not, too." We can't hear for sound now, he thinks to himself.

"Could we drive to Refugio?" she asks. "I like the name better than El Capitán."

Of course she does; he *knows* that. *Asylum, refuge, cloister,* these are her words, her constructions. "Tell me," he says, "about your childhood. You've heard too much of mine already."

"I think I've heard a lot about Sadie, but not about you alone."

He doesn't think this particularly true, but he's interested that she makes a distinction. Years ago, after someone had teasingly said to him, "Ah, yes, the gospel according to Luke here!" he'd done some research. And that Luke, the biblical Luke, had been a physician long before Luke had, and he'd written the Gospel and some of the Acts of the Apostles, and he'd written stories that no one else had told, Jesus in the temple as a boy, and Anna, the prophetess who proclaimed baby Jesus the Messiah, and he'd written them in the first person, Luke's reference insisted, the first person. But when Luke read the Bible, there was hardly ever an *I*, rarely a first-person pronoun that he could see. There was usually *we*, there was often *us*. Later, he learned it was called a "collective first person"—*we, us, our*. He thought that this was right, that the true first person was abnormally subjective—the definition of autism, he notes—and could not be a Gospel, in the sense that the Gospels were about the life of someone else, about someone's birth and death and Resurrection.

So, "No," he has to insist, and he hopes not too sternly, "Sadie's and my childhood is really not divisible. I don't suppose anyone lives outside of relation to others."

"Artists?" she asks.

"No," he says quickly, "though the best artists don't ask for confirmation from others, don't need it, probably wouldn't hear it if it arose, but they're very much in relation to others, dependent relation."

Luke looks at Alice's hands, sees them squeeze more tightly into themselves. He's always blowing it with her, being too adamant, jerky, a stereotypical doctor, a fucking steamroller. "But I'm no artist," he adds flatly. "So don't listen to me."

"I guess I believe in things that try to impart something," she says. Her right hand rises abruptly and starts to fiddle with the top button of her shirt. "Maybe I'm too much of a girl not to?"

Whoa, Luke thinks, That is a loaded couple of sentences. He supposes he understands she thinks women—girls?—necessarily more driven to communicate, or wired that way, or something. He tends to find these pop distinctions a lot of crap, perversely hopeful rationalizations for our bad behavior. If anything, he's inclined to believe that girls have a harder time getting listened to than boys and thus must work harder to communicate, but that's a pop hypothesis, too, and he doesn't want to fence on this stage built of bubble-gum wrappers. "I assume almost any serious artistic production is a will to communicate," he says, "even if just to oneself."

His words hang in the close air of the car. Maybe it's a bit stuffy. He reaches for the climate control, punches it down a few degrees. "Are you comfortable?" he asks.

"More than any human being has a right to be," she says, laughing, and he hears her saying "Cowboy dog" and laughing then, too. She's happy; he's sure of it. She likes the car. She likes riding in it, urging their way up the coast. Maybe she has a bit of that awe people have around doctors. He'll take it right now; he's not proud. He'll take her as impressed as he can get her. She has a beautiful nose and cheekbone. Already he's in love with her profile. He thinks she is one of those women who could wear her hair very short, that it would just make her bones look finer. He likes that delicate angularity, muses on that phenomenon of women—in the movies, he admits—who have been tarred and feathered or imprisoned, who are shorn of hair—how much more beautiful they appear in the extremity of their circumstance. But there is no extremity of circumstance now, no dire need, not of him, nor of rescue. *That*, he says to himself, is called "old-fashioned melodrama," or it's the movies.

"What time do you get up tomorrow morning?" he asks her, and when the question is already in the car, waiting for an answer, he realizes it sounds provocative, suggestive. It's a bit precipitous to be batting bedroom eyes. He feels the size of a moose, the huge rack and muzzle and dewlaps scrunched inside the car. Christ. A second ago, he'd actually been proud of himself for coming up with a question that wasn't about her family, for thinking through her day enough to understand that she went to the flower market very early in the mornings. Now it sounds as though he's plotting when he can fuck her, and yet when she begins to answer, it doesn't seem as though she's taken his question that way.

"About three A.M. usually. Janey and I get down there around four, when it opens. It's always dark, and I love that. It's one of the great strangenesses of the world, a flower market at four or five in the morning, all these bright flowers in darkness—at least I find there's something surreal about it, like it's underwater. Do doctors ever have time to do anything but work? Because you should come some morning and see it. You should come on a Friday, that's when the flowers are most magnificent, for the weekend."

It's pathetic, Luke thinks, what it took to get that morning free, when he'd gone down to her studio, or loft, or whatever she calls it. He could not ask a colleague to cover at St. John's, could not bring himself to say what he wanted the time for, could not cancel private appointments, or buff and turf out to someone else the consultations at Kaiser. He knows plenty of M.D.s who take a day every week, Wednesday golf day, but he's never done it, never structured his work around any type of play. He can fill a week with two weeks' worth of appointments, and now this stuff with inclusion in the public schools—mainstreaming autistics—which he thinks is its own version of insanity, but which he's nonetheless helping to write literature on, because, God knows, those teachers are going to need help! He'd love to see the flower market, and with Alice, and in the dark blue-black of morning. But he needs his sleep, so when? Then he feels old for thinking about sleep, needing it, guarding it, particularly since it's been so many months since he's had sex with someone—and really maybe it's over a year—not that he wants to contemplate that now, in this early . . . Early what, Luke? Early flowering of a relationship! And he's almost good-natured with himself, even lets the word *relationship* slide without much snideness because he recognizes the blunt physical sadness of a body that hasn't been touched, his body now, and it's not in the groin, this physical sadness; it's in the bones, and in his shoulders and in his lungs, as though someone else's touch opens all the places where the oxygen should be, should really be. . . .

"I suppose it's good to live so close to the market," he says. "You're right there already, aren't you?" and then he realizes this question or observation is suggestive, too.

"You're pretty geographically undesirable," she laughs.

He looks across the car at her, his eyes completely off the road. He's aware of cars on all sides, how dangerous it is for him to be looking at her. "I can handle geography," he says, "just as long as everything else is in the running," and when he sees that she's smiled, his eyes dart back to the road and they pass beneath a huge looming highway sign and all cars seem exactly where they were before he chanced to fix his eyes on her. "Do you think of that as what you do?" she then asks out of the blue. "Listening? Or that you're an auditor of sorts? What we were talking about earlier—you strike me as so much more willful, as a doctor, I mean."

He's never thought to use the word *auditor*—the Internal Revenue Service seems to own it—but he realizes that it's the perfect word for what he does, and for the government, too, particularly if one is paranoid and thinks Uncle Sam is always watching. His life is already different with her in it, and though he doesn't much care for the analogy that arises with the word *auditor*, he knows that observation is never far from surveillance, that listening is never far from eavesdropping, that accounting for a child's behavior might be called "diagnosis." It might as fairly be called "sentencing." None of this is new to him, these acknowledgments. What is new is how mildly he feels about it, now, in this moment.

"I don't think we've managed to hear what goes on inside an autistic child's head, or to hear the various ways in which they might attempt to communicate. In fact, when we make mistakes in therapy, when we misread them or when we don't understand them quickly enough, that's when we learn the most—when we're tumbled from our construction of the therapeutic process and are forced to see theirs. Then we make strides."

"You care a lot about your work, don't you?" she says.

Luke manages to not utter the self-serving and pathetic thought in his mind—My work is all I have—but it's kicking on the brink of his lips, about to toss itself into the world like a braying jackass. "Only Luke is with me," he quotes to himself.

"What I do at my office or at St. John's doesn't seem to me very different from just working to be sentient, responsive. Autistics are very complex people, like most people who are worth listening to—worth trying to hear."

The signs for Refugio State Beach appear and Luke exits and drives into the public parking area. It's late in the day and it's March and the lot and the beach are almost entirely empty. He parks so that they can look straight out at the ocean, but he wants to get out of the car, to walk on the beach. He wants to touch her there on the sand, to start the intricacy of any relationship they might have amid the vast possibility of the sand and the water and the air. "Shall we?" he asks, and then he changes his tune. "Get those shoes off—" And he's out of his loafers and out of the car and into the sand before she's thought to move.

His feet are happy in the lovely soft sand, which is working its cool way up between his toes. He gazes at her through the windshield. Her head is down and she is working at something in the footwell. He stands with the car remote, waiting for her to open the door and then close it and then move toward him. When she finally does, he pushes the button for the door locks and pockets the keys and works not to seem too utterly ebullient, though that's how he feels. He takes her hand in his and it is curled in upon itself in its usual way, and so he raises her hand before him and uncurls her fingers and laces his fingers into hers.

"I'm sorry," she says, and his heart torpedoes, and he supposes he must let her have her hand back, that he's been too bold too fast, and there's an eternity of consternation before she says, "I was trying to hide my purse, but I think it's probably better if we put it in the trunk. You don't need a broken-out windshield."

After he's stumbled back from his momentum, gotten himself out of the undulant sand and said, "of course, you're right, I could do without a broken window," after the remote has yipped and yacked the doors, and the purse is stowed in the trunk, and his excitement is pruned back to a proper sedate hedge, Alice reaches over and takes his hand and insinuates hers into his. It makes him look down, first at her face, her fine nose, then out across the sand. In the offing, the sky is a beautiful late-afternoon color. The color of he does not know what, but a color, he thinks. He wants to say thank you, knows he can't, knows it would sound foolish. But that's how he feels, grateful, overweeningly grateful, if the truth be told. Sadie is there, walking in front of him, marching! Her placid corduroy jumper moves about her knees like a luffless sail. She is screaming and gesturing wildly, as she will always be there screaming, gesturing wildly, her hands avid in the air at some frantic writing, and his head jerks up, because even after twenty-one years he needs to gather her in his gaze, a checking that is never casual, even now, today, as Sadie dims before him in the dense color of the sky.

"She'd be making my mother crazy—this was before they put her on Prolixin—so I'd drive Sadie to the beach that last year. Three, sometimes fours days a week—I had my driver's license finally. I'd sit back here on the sand, and if there weren't many people, I'd smoke pot and watch the ocean, and her—I'd watch her. She'd be sort of frantic for a while and then something reached her, some resource she found here, and she'd quiet and then settle in the sand, close to the water and I'd have to watch that she didn't just let herself be carried away. She didn't fear the water, and she didn't seem to get cold, even though most times she rode back home completely soaked. Maybe that's why I like my car so much; it never has wet sand in it."

Luke thinks this is truer than he would like it to be. And if he were going to allow it right now, he would hate himself a little for this thought, but he's not. He wants Alice to ask him if he ever thought of just letting the water take Sadie, of watching it wash farther and farther up the sand. It's another sentimental thought, but he wants to argue with the voice in his head, to say it's not sentimental when you know the way she did die—this would have been better, this immense saline sac. He thinks he would not mourn her death quite so much—he doesn't care that he's being romantic, or somehow mythical or allegorical. She would have died hearing something that calmed her, that took her in as its own.

He'd once been so stoned, he did let the water close all around her—or at least he didn't react until she sat entirely skirted by the tide. Then he'd raced across the sand, horrified at himself, a horror that quickly, too quickly, became his fury at her, which he supposes now has never died. "I never hit her," he says to himself, and then he sees the look of concern on Alice's face and realizes he's said this aloud. They are trudging through the sand, their feet kicking up drifts of it, and the wind is carrying it away. The air is bright and insistent, and it whirls about them, incisive, able. Alice's small deft hand is in his—completely surrounded by his—and he is talking about Sadie? All the jokes, he thinks, all the "Physician, heal thyself"s seem to swirl for a minute as she pulls her hand from his.

"And so what if you did hit her," Alice says quietly. Her dark hair has blown across her face and she reaches her hands up to brush it aside. "It must have been impossible to have Sadie as a sibling. You were a child yourself."

Luke's first inclination is to argue with her, to say, No, it was not impossible. She just *was* my sibling, and we did whatever it took, and she could be very funny and she was always right about how absurd things were in the world. But he does not argue. Instead, he just speaks what's always there, always the impossible, and at once the day-to-day reality, the facts of what happened in cut-and-dried terms. "I am still so angry that she could mask her body's messages so thoroughly, that she could take in so much, could comment on almost everything around her, but she couldn't feel her appendix bursting—I mean, how does a person get themselves in such a predicament? How do you so remove yourself from your body that excruciating pain is nothing, is like a funny tickle that makes your leg move up and down?"

Luke stops, out of breath, his anger racing. "And then how's that for the milk of human kindness—I want my sister to have felt such horrible pain that she would have had to have alerted us. That's vanity taken to another level, you must admit."

He stops talking, struggling not so much to catch his breath as to curb the momentum of his telling. He is anguished and sad and afraid of crying. He wants it all told now, today, so they can go on—if she will go on. "I think," he continues, but slowly, "I think if we knew when we were young what we'd end up wanting or desiring in later years, we might call it off pretty quickly. I'm never surprised enough by teenage suicides. Or by women who kill their children. I wonder if they're particularly prescient, if they've seen the future and that's what they can't be an accomplice to."

The waves crash toward them—at them—and Luke looks out again over the water into the dense, complex color of the horizon. He wants Alice's hand back in his own, and, of course, what he's just done is launch into the world words that can't be responded to. What the fuck is she supposed to say to that, Luke? And indeed she's not saying anything, and he reaches for her hand, and it is good in his, cool, and precious, he thinks, because he knows what her hands make, wants them on his body, around his forehead, knows somehow they remake him now in this moment with their touching. "What color would you say that is?" he asks, jerking his chin toward the water. Her face looks finely chiseled in the graying marmoreal light. He wants to watch that smooth, poreless face beneath him, his penis deep in her mouth, pushing up against the ridged palate that he knows is between her teeth. You've got me, he will say to her pulling out and then pushing slowly back in, you've got me, he will say with overwhelming desire.

She doesn't answer his question, just gazes out to sea, and then they're past the time when the question needs answering—or the answer is already indefinably between them, unspoken, articulate, the sense that derives *of* two, is suspended between two, and only survives, Luke supposes, as the two survive.

"Live with me," he blurts out, and the word *live* is not about beginnings, fresh starts, first couplings, moving in. It's about duration. It's necessary for him to be past initiation, courtship. He's not afraid of what he understands prosperous eligible men are supposedly afraid of: commitment, monogamy, financial abridgement. Whatever, he thinks with dismissal, whatever. His desperation has to do with care. Can he care enough, and properly? "Live with me," he says again, and it is precisely what he wants to say, what he wants to happen.

She looks surprised and amused and shocked and serious. "Well, you don't date," he adds, and she bursts out laughing, and he knows her belongings, whatever they are, will come to be among his. "Earthly effects," he hears Sadie scoffing. What other EFFECTS would you have! I leave my favorite chair in heaven to you—some will that would be! He sees the *Sandersonia* floating above his desk's papers and files, Alice sitting in the backyard. He starts to say, There's another room, which you didn't see, which can be your office, or the room that is your room, but he doesn't say it, doesn't need to say it. He can see in her eyes she's already there in the house, which has never seemed actually his until this moment, this very real anticipation of it being theirs, this color in the offing.

"How very old-fashioned you are, Luke," she says, and he's unhappy that he knows what she means.

"Because I haven't made sure you're a good fuck," he says, feeling cruel, all-knowing, and he can see that if she were given to defensiveness, she might balk in this moment. Instead, she apologizes, which he doesn't want, either. "What you do in the world makes me happy," he says, "very happy. And there's something you understand about care," he adds. "Or maybe nurture or sanctuary. Succor. You don't seem to like my words for it, but I trust it, you."

She turns to him, plants herself in front of him, the darkness of her hair significant against the transporting haziness of the ocean.

"My name is Alice," she states. "Alice."

Yes, he thinks, yes, I know this. Your name is Alice, and then with some weariness he understands what she might be stopping to make him see, whom she thinks she's staying his attention upon, but he does see her, does smell the mingle of ocean and perfume, smoked salmon and onion bagel, does know the small, hardworking hands in his own, the crescents of smooth dark hair about her face. There's no confusion in his mind or heart, even if Janey thinks so, his mother, others. Sadie was his sister, a girl child whom he loved as a child, a sister, whose medical and psychiatric care he regrets, indeed, has fashioned a life, a career against. A century ago, that might have been considered laudable, even noble, but now, of course, his passion is pathologized, reduced to cause and effect, questionable motivation, as though all human action were performance rather than endurance, existence. If there's any residual from Sadie, any residual that bears on his life with women, it's that he understands the treacherous difference between playacting and expertise, between sufferance and care. At sixteen, he knew about drugs, a lot about drugs, but he knew about them in the context of play, bluster, diversion; he was no expert, though he'd tried to pass himself off as such; and, of course, he'd been an expert on his little sister, Sadie, that silly dance she'd adopted of late, more high spirits from the difficult child.

He's no expert on this woman named Alice, nor is he willing to go through all the rehearsals that then, supposedly, render him sensible of their future together. He realizes he's the one who doesn't want to date. He wants to live with her, to come to a sentience of her available only through experience, and he doesn't see why they shouldn't start now, today. As far as he's concerned, he's had many months to think about this life they might live within, together. "I don't confuse you with anyone," he says, and he can't quite keep the exasperation from his voice. "I presume that's what you're suggesting. You don't stand in, replace, console any loss of my early life. I'm in love with the mind and hands that make what you make." He looks down into her face. "I like you—"

"You don't know—"

"—and don't say 'You don't know me,' because that's a silly thing to say. I can't imagine ever presuming I knew someone. I've learned that lesson," he says. "But what I experience of you, I like. What I've learned from doing what I do is that expertise is not necessarily care of an individual—so I would never say I know you. What the fuck could that possibly mean other than I've turned off enough sensors to be on the road to disaster?"

"You wouldn't, would you?" she says solemnly. "Presume, I mean," and he sees that she is nudging together a mound of sand so that she stands higher and higher before him.

He likes that she would pay him this compliment right now, that she's not insisting on quips, sallies, the great wit of legendary courtship. She feels smaller in his arms than he expected, but more intensely solid, too, the surprising liquid weight of a beaded dress his mother once handed him to take to the cleaner's—it's that weight. He finds himself already hungry for her smell, this reality of her that is so new to him, last night, this morning. It is specific and particular in this vast saline air. The day he'd visited the studio, sweet pea scented the air, and the sprightly dirt smell of damp cement, and then there was the bland Naugahyde scent of water spritzed through plastic—no smell that was Alice—but now, now she's in his lungs, a complicated richness.

They travel back toward Santa Barbara, through Isla Vista, Goleta, and then they're past Santa Barbara, Montecito, Carpinteria, names Luke loves forming in his mouth, speaking, Ventura, Montalvo, El Rio, the bounty of syllables the bounty of California, of groves and vineyards and orchards, of the ocean, and then of vast expanses of land, and the movies, those expanses of the imagination, of possibility. He likes the sexy fertility of California, so different from the matronly fecundity of the Midwest with her colossal laps of wheat. He likes California's Babylonian intricacy, dates and almonds, apricots, pistachios, peaches; he likes this harem of crops and the seduction it offers, and he likes thinking, now, in this car, smelling strawberries near Camarillo, that Alice works within this garden, and that certainly this is part of his desire. "An Angelena," she had told him on the beach, "always here."

"Never there?" he asked, looking across the sand. "Never traveled?"

"Nope," she said, like a kid, satisfied, happy. "Why—" she asks him now, in the car, "why don't you tell the real cause of Sadie's death to most people?"

Soberly, after a few beats, he asks, "How do you know that?" but he knows how she knows—Janey—and she says, "Janey," and the echo seems oddly comforting, though it shouldn't be, should, in fact, suggest he be self-conscious, sheepish, on view for lying. But just now, he's not willing to be; he wants the air she is within his lungs; he wants what she brings to the airless room called Sadie. "Did you know the real story before I told you?" he asks. "Or at least some of it?"

"Yes. I suppose I'm sorry to tell you that if you'd said leukemia or a car accident, I'd have known you were being ambiguous."

"That's a forgiving way of putting it," Luke says. "Ambiguous. Others call it evasive, or lying, or equivocation, or hiding from the truth. But then again, that's what you understand, Alice Samara, isn't it? You understand asylum."

He looks across at her and she is once again turned in her seat and gazing at him seriously. "Maybe you understand more about what I do than I do," she says frankly. "But I hear your name in the word *leukemia*, and that doesn't seem so evasive to me."

Luke feels the steering wheel in his hand, its polished wood; he feels his body suddenly afire and a weird rushing in his forehead. "No one's ever gotten that before," he says. "No one's ever heard my name in *leukemia* or *leucocytes*."

"Are you sure of that?" she asks. "You're not the last person on earth with sensibility—and believe me, I'm not the sharpest knife in the drawer, so others have gotten it. I know I don't understand your reticence about your sister."

Luke repeats the word *reticence*.

"It also strikes me that you've been carrying this around for an awfully long time.

"So, fine," he says, "you don't approve of me. I kept my mother from acting on her instincts," he adds, and there are hot coals on his heart as he tells her. "If I hadn't kept reassuring her, if I hadn't kept telling her what I knew about the drugs Sadie was on, what they would do, how they'd affect her, how long she'd sleep, how out of it she'd be, my mother would have alerted the doctors sooner, gotten her to the hospital in time."

"You seem so very sure of that," Alice says, and then she twists in her seat and sits up and asks, "Where was your father?"

"What?" Luke says a little too anxiously, but he is willing himself to calm down. "What do you mean, where was my father?"

"Just that."

"My father was gone a lot on digs," he says. "He was an archaeologist—a pre-Columbian specialist on the Manta region in Ecuador—you already know that. He also had a Ph.D. in anthropology."

"And so he wasn't there when your sister died."

"He was a great grant writer. No, he wasn't there."

Luke does feel strangely flummoxed now, confused. He realizes in his images of those days that the population includes his father, and maybe that's fairly accurate, and yet he wasn't there; he came back and forth, teaching at UCLA and then away—but back immediately upon hearing about Sadie. My father wasn't there, was he? Luke asks himself, but he knows he wasn't, just as he knows they had no dog, that a dog taking a "whiz and a bang" was just an expression his father used for all the dogs in the neighborhood, the few that wandered onto their front lawn and that his father watched studiously in order to make the distinction—"whiz!" or "bang!"—or to proclaim the bounty of both. Luke had used the expression "a whiz and bang" some time back, the words just springing to mind, but from where, he hadn't remembered.

"No," Luke says again, "no, he wasn't there on that day," and Luke sees himself standing in front of the house, the ambulance in the drive, and than another ambulance, and then the coroner, and Sadie coming out the front door so small beneath the sheet, almost not there on the gurney as it was pushed down the flagstone walk and mired for a moment in the gravel. A medic appeared and helped, and then she was slid so briskly into the coroner's van, Luke thought maybe it hadn't happened, that she wasn't there behind the beige wagon doors closing so solidly in the Sunday quiet of Brentwood. He waited on the steps as the two ambulances pulled around the circle drive and then the coroner's wagon made its way past, and Luke can see the driver nodding solemnly to him, and then holding his finger up off the steering wheel, a simple salute in recognition of what he carried in his vehicle's bay.

"You were a kid, Luke, a kid when this happened, and so what if you were smart and your mother trusted you—you still don't know if your sister would have been saved. No one can know that."

The stoplight at Kanan Dume will come up soon enough, and Luke wants for them to have something to eat in the Malibu colony. He's uncomfortably hungry, the stomach acids of anxiety. "I know you need an early night," he says, "but would you like some dinner in Malibu?"

"You would prolong this?" she asks, meaning her questioning, his sadness, which she can see she's provoked. He doesn't assume that she understands he's never out and out told anyone what he just told her in simple, exacting terms. Not even when he was being shrunk did he tell the entire truth about his complicity; that's how good he is with telling other stories. But now he wants to talk about them, to come back to the subject of their future—if they have a future.

"I trust what unfolds in time, Alice, more than I trust what arises suddenly in speed."

"Luke, you just asked me to live with you. Few would consider that a long engagement."

"What I mean," he says, "by unfolding in time is us unfolding in time. Let's not start from some arbitrary demarkation— an engagement, marriage, a first fuck—let's not start there as though from *that* we're suddenly miraculously right for each other. Who the fuck knows? All that cheering and congratulating, and for what? No one's left the starting gate."

The car is silent, disastrously so, he thinks, and then his car phone rings. He doesn't know whether to resent this intrusion or to breathe easier because it affords him hang time. "Excuse me," he says hoarsely. In his ear, Jordan Markens speaks quietly, quickly, apologetically, excitedly—he can hear she doesn't exactly know which note to strike. "I know it's Sunday, and I'm sorry to disturb you. I know it could have waited, but Polly just did something very unusual."

"Unusual for Polly?" he asks.

"She just dressed up in a worm costume."

"Really?" Luke says, incredulous. "A costume?"

"And then she went downstairs and showed Stewart."

"Did you make a bit of a big deal over it?" he asks. "Did Stewart?" Jordan Markens laughs, and it's a sound Luke has never heard before, low and throaty, maybe a laugh learning once again to be about happiness, joy.

"Doctor, I'm not the one who has trouble showing affect. I was practically hysterical."

"Did she role-play at all?" he asks. "You know, did she take on another character?" Because the road has become particularly curvy, Luke slows the car by disengaging the clutch and braking rather than downshifting. He doesn't like when the phone prevents him from driving, the free float of the car released from the secure pull of gears. "Jordan, may I put you on the speaker phone?" he asks. "Someone's with me, though. I just want you to know that. A friend. We're driving into Malibu."

"No," Jordan Markens says, "I don't mind—my child's not a state secret. Can you believe it, Doctor?"

Luke apologizes to Alice and replaces the headset. "I just want a few more details while they're fresh," he says, taking the stick shift into his hand and moving it snugly, rightly into first. "A persona, Jordan? Any sort of suggestion of another character?" he asks again. "She act worm-like, even?" He listens carefully for any change of inflection in Jordan's voice. His questions cause some parents to feel that he is testing them, putting their actions on display, when all he wants is for them to be his ears and eyes, to be as an adept an observer as they can possibly be.

"No," Jordan Markens says, "no, she didn't. She just stood there quietly." But Luke hears that there's no force in the world that can keep the hope from Jordan's voice right now. "She did put on this costume completely of her own accord, Doctor. That is good, isn't it?"

"It's very, very good," Luke states, and he's immensely happy to be able to utter these words, to mean them, though he rarely, if ever, pacifies a parent. Sometimes he longs to write a prescription and to hear a few days later that an infection is gone, a wound healed. "Jordan," he says, "this may be logistically difficult, but can you pay a lot of attention to Polly right now? Stay close to her, talk to her a lot, you know, just really try to keep her in your sights, in your focus, if possible. Can you keep her focused outward as much as you can?"

Jordan's voice sounds suddenly more quiet in the car. Luke thinks perhaps Polly has come into the room where she is, or Stewart, one of the other three children. "Yes, okay, sure."

Luke has an idea. "Jordan, are you about to cook dinner?"

"We were taking the kids for pizza."

"Let Stewart go, and why don't you and Polly stay home—you can order a pizza in. Could that happen?" Luke is acutely aware of Alice listening to him, and equally aware of putting Jordan Markens in a position with her husband. Stewart Markens is no honey bear. "Jordan, just do what you can to keep a bit of focus on Polly, okay, and I'll see you tomorrow."

"Thank you, Doctor, and I'm sorry to have disturbed your Sunday."

"You've made my Sunday, believe me, you have. Maybe my friend and I will have pizza, too." He pushes the off button on the headset, is markedly aware of his arm for some reason, his male arm stretching out across the cab of the car, the scale of his arm so different from that of Alice's, a sort of wondrousness about its size. He starts to say something to Alice, to suggest some restaurants—God knows there's no decent pizza in this town—but she stops him. "I think I understand, and I think I'm beginning to understand something about you, why you're good at what you do, your comment about time. You know your friends who hired me for that christening you went to, the doctors—they called the other day for flowers for a shower and I told them I'd met you. I understand from them that you're a little famous. You have a case study published somewhere? A success story, I guess? A boy and something about electrical machines he made to run himself on—or that you realized he needed and so helped to build."

"I'm a little famous *within the field*, please, and I would never have gotten as far *as quickly* as I got with Emmett without the wisdom of many doctors before me, and one case, somewhat similar, and very well documented, which aided me greatly because the interpretive skills of the therapist were so brilliant, but if you want, I'll give you an offprint to read. I treated Emmett for six years, it's true, and he attends Brown, and maybe he wouldn't if it weren't for me, but maybe he would, too? Autistics are very powerful in their own way. Maybe I nurtured his access to that power—that's the only conscionable way to state it. He'll still have a lot of trouble in the world, always, and he'll probably never have a romantic relationship. Many aspects of life you and I just take for granted, think of as our right, he'll never enjoy, and, what's perhaps even worse, will never be able to understand why not."

"I'd like that."

She'd like what? A life without romantic love? Dinner? And then he realizes she'd like to read the case study. He thinks the offprints from the *Journal of Autism and Developmental Disorders* are in one of the boxes he stashed in the garage this morning in preparation for her arrival, a somewhat tall, narrow box, which he can see in his mind's eye shoved up onto a shelf next to the liquid sulfur his mother gave him for whitefly. Isn't it interesting this article should come up, that he's just had his hands on the copies? He supposes these publications should not really be in the garage, though the garage is watertight.

"What about the other, both immediate, as in dinner, and tomorrow, as in 'How about it?' I promise dinner will be short."

"Short," she says, "short dinner—"

"Long life?"

"We'll see, Luke. We will just have to see."

That is not what he wants to hear right now. He slows the car into second around a particularly tight curve. He feels as though he's pulling himself into lower and lower gears, slowing himself down all the way to a halt so that he can throw himself into reverse, but what did he expect? "Logistics are bad, aren't they?" he asks. "You're set up down there; you're near the flower market, you live within your warehouse garden. It's perverse of me even to want you to move, isn't it?"

"Oh yes, crass and brutish. If it's okay with you," she says slowly, "I'll read your asking me to move in with you as your desire, not your perversity. When someone claims perversity it's an affectation. Real perverseness doesn't announce itself."

He's somewhat unnerved by this perception, which seems more like something he'd be the expert of. A typical person using the word *perverse* casually—well, God knows what he or she might mean. But he hadn't really used *perverse* in the vernacular, either. Something did seem normal, right, all of a piece, Alice Samara a cloistered figure at the center of her life— this was right, wasn't it! And what he wanted drove against it, threatened to mangle it.

"You like oysters?" he asks.

"I do—"

"Thank fucking God, a woman who likes oysters."

Luke doesn't usually hear himself swear, but he does now, the words bluntly acid, dull, unnecessary, and silly in their severity because unnecessary.

"Cussing a blue streak," she says, as though she knows to diffuse the moment, even to let him save face.

"Profanity bother you?" he asks.

"Of course not."

"Somehow it fits the tenor of the age."

"You mean the tenor of Luke."

"Perhaps," he says. "But we don't live outside of time, an age."

"Sometimes we do, don't we? Your sister died of something almost no one dies of today. That seems outside of present time."

Mountains outlined in the bright dimness of twilight rise on either side of the car. The canyon deepens as they descend to the ocean. Luke does not want to go on, to dinner, or anywhere. He has made a mistake about this love of his, and the coarse, uncomfortable beat of his heart tells him so. It's one thing to let someone in this airless room called Sadie; it's quite another to have them rearrange the furniture. He is willing to take blame, even to place blame, as he has recently learned, on his mother, maybe even his father, but he's not willing to have futility be the complexion of Sadie's death. CHILD DIES BECAUSE RELIGIOUS PARENTS REFUSE THE GODLESS ARM OF SCIENCE, some simplistic story like that. All Sadie had needed was an appendectomy, that was true, at least all she needed for that particular bit of infection, but *you have to understand*, he's desperate to say, she was dancing, laughing—she had the best medical care money can provide. And then he does say, "She was dancing, you know, maybe I've told you that? She was sick and she was being treated for it, psychosis, schizophrenia, but the night before she died, she was doing a kind of jig in my doorway—she was on her way to bed."

"But it wasn't, was it?"

"No, it wasn't," and Luke doesn't know whether he wants to shout this at her, to continue to claim this ancient anguish, or to set the words behind him, as though they are a structure of the past, some brooding scaffolding that spells out *it wasn't a jig* and which he nows walks out from under.

"It's something . . ." she says slowly, "something that I haven't really thought about for years. I don't think I ever told anyone about it, either, and my brother wasn't there, didn't see it. I don't think he knows—strange how children grow up together but almost in parallel universes. Your question in the studio that day annoyed me, about Hiroshima. It seemed strange, or some wildly constructed, overcooked pickup line, and yet I couldn't figure out why you would allude then to an event so horrifying, so violent if you weren't also serious."

"I'm feeling a bit misunderstood," he says easily, trying for humor, but then he wants to talk seriously about Alice's work. "I actually find your compositions uncanny—"

"Overhearing your conversation about your patient. Polly? Is that her name? Polly?"

"Yes," he says, "Polly."

"I remembered, I mean, not that I'd forgotten, but I realized what it was you were seeing, I mean I guess what you're seeing, not the event, not what happened, but what I did."

"What did you do?" he asks.

"I ran."

"You were afraid . . ." he says.

"That my father would punish me, and so I ran, and I hid—"

"To protect yourself." He glances at her quickly, then pulls his eyes back to the curving road, the canyon unfurling toward sea level, highway, ocean.

"That's strange," she says, "because that's what would make sense, but no, I didn't try to protect myself, or I did, but not really. I ran behind our house into the chaparral, where there were huge bushes of poison oak, and I knew they were poison oak, but that's where I hid myself."

At the end of the canyon, just ahead, is Pacific Coast Highway. Luke can see the red of the stoplight, and cars speeding past along the coast, streaks of red, streaks of white. He is lodging the stick shift into lower and lower gears, using the engine to slow the car but keeping the tac up, blipping the gas. He's acutely aware of driving, his body coolly working the car. "Poison oak is very, very beautiful," he says, coaxing, trying not to. "What time of year was it, because in the fall the leaves are particularly beautiful, colored. You're not the first—"

"No," she says adamantly. "I knew what poison oak was, what it caused. I was hospitalized. I couldn't open my eyes for almost three weeks."

"What had you seen?" he asks.

"Maybe just what a lot of children have seen."

"It's not a contest."

"Spend the night with me," she says. "When we get my car, we can get you some clothes. You don't have a pet."

"And you do," he says.

"He must have been with the dog walker when you were at the loft."

"Dog walker? Let me guess, you also hire a bodyguard for the dog walker?"

"That's right," she says, "dog walker bodyguard." The sound of her saying "Cowboy dog" fills his ears and he recalls the lanky brown dog bounding about her legs at the gas station. "Cowboy dog" must have smelled Alice's dog on her, but he doesn't really want this pheromonal explanation, prefers to just see the dog's leaping, bounding excitement unconnected to science, biology, one beast sniffing out another, as Luke is no doubt doing right now, carefully aware of his breathing, of what's in the air of his nose, the power beneath his hands at the behest of his arms and legs. She's leaned forward in her seat and he can see just past the collar of her shirt to her skin, to the edge of lace along a bra strap, to a thin gold chain he didn't know she wore. "Anything on the end of that chain?"

"He's a Bouvier," she says. "I call him Jack—short for Jacqueline Bouvier Kennedy." She holds out from her chest a small orb of turquoise that seems to have been grooved in spirals. He looks from the orb back to the red light at Kanan Dume. He wants to reach across and feel the warmth of this bauble that has hung there all day between her breasts.

"Most people who get that find it funny," she says after awhile. "Jacqueline Bouvier Kennedy." There's no prickliness in her voice.

It is funny, and he has thought to laugh, but somehow just hasn't. He says this, says he wants to spend the night with her, says that they can do food any number of ways. "Here are some proposals." And as he starts to run variables, cold shrimp and lobster to take downtown, or sushi, or oysters looking out over the Pacific, she stops him with her small hand on his knee. Its heat seems heavy, molten. She is so startling, he thinks, the intensity of her size, like lead shot or a baby's head. "You won't starve," she says. "Just come to my place. I'll take care of things," and then her hand lifts—is gone—his knee cooling. How unusual it is for him to hear the details of someone's life . . . and to have almost nothing expected of him save affection, audition. What she had run from was either something very small, maybe something not even disturbing to an adult, or something so ugly that describing it was impossible. But he would wait as long as was needed, and she would tell him simply, and in clear language—and it wouldn't be because he was a doctor.

She backs down his driveway, the toss of her dark hair framed in the broad, straightforward window, a car window from another era, crystal clear and unfussily shaped. At least there's visibility, Luke thinks, but no automatic locks, and doors as easy peasy to get into as a jar of pickles. He doubts one would even need a Slim Jim; a paint stick would probably do just as well. Her car moves down the street, its bright orange panels flashing in the streetlights. He watches. He wants her to wave to him like she did that first day in her studio, the small hand simply raised, simply waving. Why would she wave to you, Luke? he chides himself. She's going to see you in an hour. But he can't quite believe that, either, that he will get in his car and drive downtown and pass through the gauntlet of electric eyes and that he'll then, after this trip of speed and clear passage, this trip of no hardship or barriers, that he'll then spend the night in her bed. He looks from the street, empty now of anything he wishes to see, to the ornamental pear in bloom on his front lawn. There's a solid skirt of white petals at the base of its narrow trunk. He's seeing the future, a sweet white bed and Alice leaving it for the flower market, leaving them, before it's light out.

His attention is drawn back down the block to a sports utility vehicle whose alarm has gone off unprovoked. The SUV sits there darkly, tinted windows and black paint, inanimate and shrieking. He waits, hating the absurd lack of peril within the even more absurd desperation of its alarm. He looks at his watch, starts to time the situation, an occupational habit. Empty fortress indeed, he thinks, the title of Bettelheim's book on autism, a title he's always hated, thought profoundly cruel and. worse, inaccurate. But here, *here* is an empty fortress. One minute and no one has even emerged from a house, let alone shut the thing off. He needs to gather some things, to leave a number with his service, but he's intensely interested in just how long this alarm will sound without a response. He is actually convinced Schopenhauer is right, this link between intelligence and sensitivity to sound. He feels beset by the idiotic property of the contemporary world and that world's—his world's—rage to protect this property. Could a child crying differentiate her cry enough to be heard within this mechanical shrieking?

Three—almost four—minutes before the alarm is finally shut off. Luke's standing in his bedroom, zipping a shirt into a hanging case. He turns his wrist to check the time. The instant quiet, for some reason, makes him aware of his hands, one holding the shoulder of the case, the other the zipper pull. His hands are sizable, with long fingers—he is a big man. How much trust a woman must feel before she lets herself be undressed, touched, entered. Is it a conscious decision on her part—these hands will gentle me; these hands will not strangle or maul me? He knows some women thrill to the possibility of violence, provoke the suggestion of reversal within the love- making. Alice has so easily acquiesced—that's not the right word—but she's allowed him in. He doesn't quite believe it. He will go downstairs to the basement for a bottle of champagne, or maybe a bottle of Syrah or pinot. Scotch, he remembers, taking up the handles of his leather duffel. She drinks Scotch, the glass suspended from her fingers, her fingers like a bail—and behind her his mother's tall garden walls covered with the three espaliered trees he has known most of his life. He moves to the dining room, drops the duffel at his feet, and hunkers before the sideboard. He draws out an unopened bottle of Mortlach and slides it into the duffel alongside his Dopp kit. He knows he should arrive with nothing but the scotch tucked in close to his body in a good leather coat, the collar turned up, that he shouldn't look like he's moving in, or that he cares about—what?—personal hygiene, a change of underwear. Yeah, well, he does care. He's had his days of standing in women's doorways looking cool, tall, and so looking down, looking just degenerate

enough to slacken all but the drive toward abandon. He has a
7 A.M. with L.A. County Unified, and no, Janey, he wasn't born
with a necktie on, but he sure as hell has one noosed about himself now. Change of clothes—hadn't Alice said that, hadn't that
been her idea anyway? Where the hell does the dog sleep?

The SUV alarm resumes its shrieking and then stops again,
leaving a pitched anticipatory silence, which Luke also resents,
because even though the thing isn't sounding off, he's now waiting for it to shriek again. Its silence owns him, too. How did we
come to care for metal so much we gave up our ears for it?

He wants one last thing and he walks to his den. The door
opening incites a breeze in the room, and when he switches on
the light, the *Sandersonia* are moving goofily over his desk. He
sits in his chair and swivels around to the case of books at his
back. He knows precisely where the thin paperback is, wedged
on its side with a purple rubber band holding its pages together,
a band that once bound broccoli stems. He coaxes the band off
and studies the mushroom cloud on its cover. It looks more like
a brain and brain stem and spinal cord; he is not the first to
remark this resemblance. He swivels back to his desk and the
book falls open in his hands. "All day, people poured into Asano
Park," he reads. "This private estate was far enough away from
the explosion so that its bamboo, pines, laurel, and maples were
still alive, and the green place invited refugees—partly because
they believed that if the Americans came back, they would
bomb only buildings; partly because the foliage seemed a center of coolness and life, and the estate's exquisitely precise rock
gardens, with their quiet pools and arching bridges, were very
Japanese, normal, secure; and also partly (according to some
who were there) because of an irresistible, atavistic urge to hide
under leaves."

He will read this to her this evening. There will be a
moment put aside within their time and he will draw *Hiroshima*
forth and recite it—because he can recite it, though he will read
it nonetheless—and he will watch her face in the dim light—it
will be dim light—and she will know why he's putting these
words in the air about them. She will tell him the story. Because

there is a story, that menace she ran from, and then a thicket of poison oak within which she cloistered and within which she still cloisters, abstracted from the past.

He can smell her in his car, feels she might still be tangibly there as he moves his hand to call his mother on his cellular, but his hand moves unimpeded, easily, and his mother's voice is soon there in the car as he drives down his street, past the black SUV, which now, uncannily, its alarm silent, seems to be brooding.

"I don't blame you," he says without salutation. "You know that, don't you?"

"Maybe, maybe not. Where are you going?" she asks.

He waits at the stoplight he thinks of as the light that lets the cars out of his neighborhood. The light is taking a long time to turn, but then again, this light always takes a long time to turn. It's Sunday evening. The streets sit quietly, anticipating, a sound stage upon which the action has not yet begun.

"Oh, I see, I see," she says merrily, because he's not answered. "And on a school night, no less!"

"What do I mean," he says slowly, "what do I mean when I say 'I never asked' about Sadie?" The words seem to hover in the dark of the car, palpable. They have a simplicity, a clearness of request. "Mom?"

"Becoming a doctor only made this worse: you had to think that you knew what had happened. That was the only way you could take responsibility for her death."

"And I was going to do that no matter what."

"Yes, it seemed to me you were going to do that no matter how senseless it was—no matter how far afield of the facts."

Something seizes at the center of his face, the bridge of his nose driven up into his forehead as though someone has punched him. "No matter how senseless Sadie's death?" he manages to ask.

"No, Luke. No matter how senseless your taking responsibility for it was."

The light turns green, but he is slow to depress the accelerator and he drives through on the yellow, which angers him:

He wants to be at Alice's or to *get* there quickly. "What did you think of last night?" he asks, not really knowing what he wants by way of an answer. "What did you think of her?" he then asks.

"Oh, I don't really think I need to weigh in about last night," Louise says. "How was your tennis game with your patient's father? I forgot to ask."

"Not good, but his son's doing better."

"He's the boy you like so much?"

"Yeah . . . that's a strange thing, isn't it?" he says. "These kids all have the experience of not being liked. That's on top of everything else." He is thinking about tomorrow morning, about autistics and public schools and the particular menace of playgrounds.

"Luke, if I'm not mistaken, you are driving off to spend the night with a woman. Why don't you—" And he hears Janey and his mother laugh, though it is gentle.

"I'll call you tomorrow," he says quickly, and then the line is quiet. He sees her in the stuffed chair in her bedroom, her hair still furled up in its French twist, though there are feathers of silver now around her neck and face because it is late. The floor is strewn about with large gardening books. Janey is there, sprawled across the bed, and her head is wrapped in plastic and stewing in whatever this week's color is.

In the darkness, the ramp coming off the 10 is somber, desolate, the tire skids along the walls catching in the car lights—there, not there—teasing, like nighttime footage in a movie. He's taking it too quickly and he has to brake, swerving around the curve. His heart pumps and then the car straightens out and he's under the freeway in its deeper petroleum darkness. The gas station is there to the right, dimly lit as he emerges from the underpass. It still reminds him of a thirties crime novel, some grimly thin existentialist piece set in the murky light of industry at rest. His car moves sleekly by. Not my setting, he thinks, not where my imagination is tonight. In a few blocks, he turns left and starts down the gauntlet of electrical gates, each with its single beady eye. He once again holds the mysterious white card the size of a credit card and yet twice as thick. She has told him to gesture it back and forth before the eyes, not to feed it through the machines as he had done that first day. Low brick buildings on either side sit darkly and there is concertina wire spiraling along their rooftops, and then there is a yard of sorts with mounds of gravel. He's having no luck with the second gate, semaphoring the card up and down, right to left, feeling a little silly, but finally the gate arm rises and he moves the car into gear and accelerates slowly past taller brick buildings through to the next gate. She's standing, waiting for him just within the door of her building, within the sharp industrial glare of several overhead lights in cages. Four gates, his arms waggling ridiculously before each aperture—but there she is standing before him once again!

"I'm going to park you inside," she says. "I've moved our van. Just drive around to the side and I'll raise the door."

"Yes, okay," Luke says, looking down at her. She has changed her shoes to flat, vaguely orthopedic clogs, shoes he would have thought she might work in. But that first day, she'd stood there—across the loft—in low black heels, that one foot propped just so on the stool rung. He passes back out the metal doors. He realizes she looks tired—is tired—can hear it in the draggy calm of her speech. He shouldn't be here. It's Sunday. She needs to be up inordinately early. He's being a doctor? He's being a human being? He doesn't really know. He sees what he sees as he hears the bolt slide into place in the door he's just let close behind him: She's exhausted. The car phone is ringing when he pulls his door open. Not what he needs right now. He needs them all to manage without his help for just a few more hours, but that's not a desire he's had for many, many years, and his arm instinctively reaches for the headset.

"Who schedules an appointment for seven o'clock in the morning?"

"Hey, Albertine," he says, relief in his voice.

"You got that," she says.

He starts his car and backs it up. "How was your weekend?"

"Fine, other than I thought to myself just a minute ago: any fool who would make an appointment at seven A.M. is fool enough to forget it, too."

Luke drives slowly around the side of the building and sees a bank of metal industrial doors and then one rolling slowly up into its cannister. "Not my choice exactly. I'll be in by nine."

"Henry's grandmother called Saturday morning. She wants to talk—"

"Can I get it all tomorrow?" Luke asks. Alice is in his headlights, her hand held over her eyes. He switches them off and pulls the car alongside a dark green van parked behind a larger truck. He realizes her business is much bigger than he's consciously allowed, that he's kept it small in his mind, and personal, not anything significant enough to thwart his plans—not a character in the dramatis personae. "Albertine?"

"Yes, I'm here."

"Thank you," he says, "I would have forgotten that appointment."

"No, you wouldn't have, but I thought I'd better make sure," she says. "See you tomorrow."

Luke hears the metal door rattling back down as he steps from his car. The loading dock smells strangely homey, as though pies are baking, cinnamon, cloves, maybe pepper, and yet the air of the dock is cold. The baking smells register on his face and she laughs. "You were expecting the scent of flowers? I thought I'd mull you some cider!"

He assumes she's joking, but he's not entirely sure, either.

"It's back on one of these loading bays. He's Czech and he's brewing—or stewing, or distilling, whatever the word—this liqueur he can't find here in the United States. Janey loves it."

"It's another world down here, isn't it?" he says.

"Yeah, well, we need visitations from the outside." She has pulled open the passenger door and retrieved his duffel. She's holding it in front of her with both hands. It's something a man would do, retrieve luggage, and he likes that she has made this practical gesture, that it's out of graciousness, hospitality. She is also—standing there—a bit kidlike, as though the favorite uncle has come to visit. He's unnerved by her unabashed affection, feels incapable of receiving it. He takes the duffel from her, but she leaves her hands attached to its straps and then her arms are around his neck and the duffel is swung across his shoulder. "What do you have in that bag?" she asks, her breath feathering across his ear.

"Scotch."

"Oh," she says sadly.

"Don't worry. I figured it out," he says. "Another time." She feels relaxed in his arms, supple, half at home already. "You are going to feed me, though, aren't you? I'm starved."

"I am," she says, dropping away from him, "I am." He watches her pull his car's back door open and grab his hanging case. "I just can't drink and get up early—or I can and then I feel shitty."

"It's all okay."

"Bark the car," she says, walking away, weaving in and around dozens of tall iron standards, arches, chuppahs, bails of chicken wire. He can see past it all to the industrial elevator and the metal box with the call button inside. She stands there now, almost completely obscured behind his case hanging down her back. *Bark the car,* and then he gets it and clicks his car remote, and it does bark, once, a quick bark, a yelp, really. He wants to keep her in his view, but he can't and make it through this course of obstacles, this thicket of standards with long metal feet ready to trip him and tumble him to the cement. He finds these wedding and party props rather conventional for her work and it surprises him to see them here, haphazard, and wildly haired with thin green florist wires, defoliated. He hears the elevator shambling down the shaft, and the clang and rattle of the grille being pulled back, and when he looks up, she stands there holding the long brass lever, waiting. "Feel better about your car?" she asks. Luke knows she is teasing and that she would normally be right, but oddly he has not once in these last few hours thought about the safety of his car. He steps into the springiness of the elevator floor, remembering this floor's ease, watches her as she slides the grille into place, watches her turn to him, his hand reaching for the turquoise bauble, his hand between her breasts, one button pulled from its hole, another, another, his hand in this preternatural heat, his lips against her neck, her cheek, her ear, her lips on his and then so many words between them, within them, within the rattling slow transport.

"Janey called me a doofus." Luke breathes the words across her cheek.

"That seems mild enough. Why?"

"I hadn't realized you lived here," he says. She is wrapped deep within his arms now, molten against his chest, and as they ascend in the shaft, it is momentarily completely dark, and then their bodies are streaked with light and then this dims. "You got to stop this rig?" he asks her. He hears voices and music playing somewhere. It's inviting, isolating. It's like a city in one of those post-apocalyptic films, the hyper-industrialized living space and within it characters making plans and cleaning futuristic weaponry beside small primordial fires. "Anything could go on down here, couldn't it?"

"Imagination running away with you, Doctor? Mostly people work here, make art—"

"Distill alcohol."

"Sure, that, too."

"Where does this dog sleep? Jack."

"Worried about meeting him?"

"Sure, as you like to say, *sure*, I'm worried about meeting the dog."

"Don't be. He likes guys a whole lot," but Luke doesn't want to hear about *guys* right now. Her back seems incredibly narrow in his hands. She knew to park his car in one of the bays. Is that because she is used to having men park their cars there, or does everyone do this because of the area?

"I'm really happy you're here," she says, and Luke is stunned by how easily she is saying this, holding so little back, in fact nothing back, as far as he can see. Perhaps Janey helped him more than he'd thought. From "doesn't date" to this? He's puzzled and a bit unhappy about other "guys," but then again, he is not going to let it stop a thing. He starts to say something, but it tangles horribly in his mouth, and because the lift is slowing and about to stop, he pretends that's why he has paused, but she isn't fooled. "You're thinking, 'Why did this time have to be so long in coming?'" she says. "Right? Just sometimes things do. You know that better than most, Luke, so don't contradict yourself." She pulls away from him, sliding beneath his arm. "Sorry to do this," she says, and there is a click and a bare lightbulb glares overhead. He can't see for a moment, but when he turns, he looks out through the grille across the warehouse space he saw months ago. He sees her work area, the small forest of ficus trees, the hose snaking across the floor. She's holding his hanging case and his bag, looking at him, and then turning to pull the grille open.

"Where exactly is it that you live?" he asks, and he reaches out—catches her, really, before she steps off the lift—and takes his bag from her. "Wouldn't want you to drop the scotch." A dog barks and Luke can hear it's a happy bark if there is such a thing, excited, gleeful. He realizes he might be jealous of a dog. Great, just great. She waits for him and then shoves the grille closed and because of the dog barking, the rattle and crash are muted. He follows her and then watches as she stops at her table and looks at a list of names with functions and notes. She works hard, struggles, he might even say. "Aren't you going to have to hire other people besides Janey?"

"I do hire other people. All of the time—who said different?" she asks, and she is the Alice of the first day he met her, far away, distracted, a little tough. "I have a staff. One person couldn't do this, not even two. You just haven't seen where they work." She leans to write something down on a tablet and he takes his other case from her. He had been under the impression that Janey was the only one who worked with her. He can now see just how little sense that makes. He had certainly clung to an idea of her as having a hobby and not a profession within which she was not only established but highly regarded. "Sorry," she murmurs, "I just need to think about this for a minute. Mondays are almost always light," and just when he thinks that she is as far away as she can possibly be, she says, "That's why you came on a Monday."

"So you remember?"

"Of course I remember. See that tree over there. There's a switch behind it. Push it and I'll be right there."

"I don't really understand," Luke says. He stands there, near her horseshoe table, not moving. "Why did it take so long? Sure, sometimes things take a long time. I know, believe me I know, but why did this take such a long time? Maybe there's something I need to know?"

"There's always something one needs to know, but I don't think it needs to be now. I'd like to finish—"

"Why not now, Alice?" Luke puts his duffel on the clean surface of her table and then drapes the hanging case over it. "Now is a good time, wouldn't you agree? Don't we have a little time right now—isn't this time that we've just given ourselves?"

The dog, Jack, barks once, and then is silent for a beat, and then he barks forcefully. Luke listens to him as he watches Alice turn in the splotchy light and look up at him. Her face is serious and calm and questioning. "You need to finish whatever you're doing," he says. "I'm being a jerk."

"This is a good thing, Luke, and I like how I am allowed this work in the world, and anything we might have together must allow this, yes?"

"Of course," he says quickly. "Of course, but that wasn't what I was getting at."

"Yes, I know, and now can you go release Jack before he's so antagonized that he bounds out of there and tries to take your leg off."

Luke walks across the floor thinking *dog*. There's a dog behind this wall frothing at the mouth, one he's not particularly keen to meet, but Luke also wants to see her living quarters. He expects a door, the switch to be for a light that illuminates a way in, a door handle, a short flight of stairs, but the switch is a metal toggle, and when he throws it, the wall slides back à la James Bond, pocketing itself as it rolls. Jack is huge and silvery black and his barking wags his entire furry body. Luke is simultaneously pleased and annoyed that Jack seems about as efficacious a guard dog as a bowl of porridge. Jack smudges Luke's knee with saliva and then circles him, barking and wagging his tail and bouncing back on his hind paws. Maybe Luke's happy about that gun after all, and when she walks in beside him, he says, "Where do you keep your gun? Handy, I hope."

She articulates the word *gulp*, and then he says to her that that would be unusual, a man using a gun on a woman in a situation like this.

"They have statistics for that sort of thing, too," she says. She is reaching into a circuit breaker box and Jack is dancing around her legs. "Wow."

"For almost everything, but what I was referring to is Jack not being much of a guard dog."

"He barks. I thought that was the most important aspect of having a dog around. Barking."

"Okay," Luke says. "Okay."

"How have I survived thus far? Amazing."

It is, Luke says to himself, it is, and he sees she has set a coffee table—really a massive piece of stone polished flat on top—with votives, which are lit and flickering, and as the wall slides back into place, he looks at the entire space, its hugeness more vertical than horizontal, the massive industrial windows high up in the walls and the light clerestorical. He sees a low bed on a white leather frame, very contemporary Italian, stacks of large art books everywhere, and a kitchen area with a trapezoidal stone counter with jagged unpolished edges—and not a lot else. It puts him immediately at ease. No bowered canopies, no doll collection, but then again, he hadn't really expected that. He hadn't expected this, either, streamlined and sleek and modern. Then again, it was L.A.

"You seem puzzled," she says. He watches her take down a single glass, a whiskey tumbler, from one of the glass cabinets along the wall of the kitchen area. It's a nice glass, Luke can see, a beautiful glass he realizes when he sets his cases down and picks it up. He fingers its smooth, sharply cut planes. He watches her lean down and tousle Jack's head and then send him to his bed, a big round dog pad, which seems the only shabby thing here. Jack seems remarkably well trained, or too used to male visitors, Luke can't keep himself from thinking.

"Do you have a knife?" he asks. "A junky one—for cutting this lead." He hauls his case up onto a chrome counter stool, sits in the other one, and pulls the bottle of Mortlach out. He doesn't want to drink alone. She is looking at him, waiting to catch his eye, but he thinks he'll not look up. She is reading him too well.

"Do you always ask for this much weaponry on your first night with a girl? And what's wrong with a lead cutter?"

"The bottle neck is too big," he says.

"Hey," she urges, "what's up with you all of a sudden?"

"You remember it was a Monday when I first came, you remember what I said, so why—"

"No, no, something else, though maybe they're connected?"

"Jack doesn't seem particularly put out by my presence."

"Want him to be? Because we can certainly make this turn on a dime."

"Was there somebody in your life when I came to visit that time?"

"Jack's not a guard dog; he's a pet. Actually, he's used to being with a lot of different people, to being down on the dock with about four delivery guys at any given time. But, Luke, I also have history, a life before you, not much of one, but *one*. You were the guy who could wait to find out, who didn't need to know a thing—remember. But no, there wasn't anyone, or at least no one in particular, and now that I've said that, you'll ask me again, why, why did it take so long. It did."

"I surprise myself even," he says slowly, "and you're not stupid enough to be flattered, so I'm looking like an ass."

"Yes, you are."

She is holding a knife out to him, the blade gingerly between her fingers, the handle suspended, waiting for him to take it. Instead, he reaches across and grabs her wrist and pulls her around the counter. With his other hand, he takes the knife handle and then holds it flat against her back. He has her pinned within his thighs, her back against the counter. He fills his lungs with her again, his face in her hair, his nose against her neck, his lips on her shoulder, her collarbone. He realizes she is alarmed, frightened, and trying not to be, but he feels it and loosens his hold, just enough so that he is running the knife blade beneath the lip of the stopper, cutting the lead. He looks across her shoulder at what he's doing, and then he drops his eyes to her face, sees her seriousness, and looks back over her shoulder. He wants to ask her who or what "Sweet pea" is, wants to see her face brighten, her eyes become alive again the way they had how many months ago when he'd said "sweet pea" walking across the floor to her, the first words he'd ever spoken in her presence, but he's just put her in a defensive place and her body is stiff, unyielding. He's not going to get her to talk now. He lets his arm drop. He pulls his leg back, and she moves away. When he looks up from pouring scotch, he realizes a pasta pot has begun to boil on the stove. It's not as early as he would like it to be, but it's not late, either. He allows himself to believe that there will be time, time that he has asked for. She's cutting sun-dried tomatoes into slivers, something he is not fond of. He likes his scotch, her standing a few feet from him, her dark hair fallen forward and then tossed back with the shake of her head. There's no music; it's quiet except for the pot rattling softly, Jack panting. She starts to apologize for the food, to say she hadn't expected company, but he stops her, shakes his head, smiles, how could I be happier, hmm, how? he asks with his eyes, and in an hour, when he is inside of her, gazing down at her beneath him, her dark hair spread out over his forearms, which encircle her head, he says aloud, "Maybe now I'm happier than I was an hour ago, maybe now." *Sweet pea* he says in his mind, *sweet pea*, the arch of her eyebrow a perfect feather. "Sweet pea," he intones, and then she looks up and very quietly says, "It was the nurse, in the hospital, who took care of me, three weeks of changing sheets soaked in pus. She called me sweet pea."

"Well, now the doctor is here," he says, and the words are out in the air before he thinks, before he hears Louise cautioning him, but then, as so often it seems with Alice, it's all fine, it's a small joke shared in their first bed, and sweet pea is now already his word for her, words he supposes, words. He recites to her from memory the passage from *Hiroshima*.

"'An irresistable, atavistic urge.' That about describes now," she says, and he can feel her stomach rolling with amusement, laughter. "I don't think that has much to do with me hiding in poison oak."

"I've always been struck by the detail of the leaves, what people might seek fleeing atrocity, and when I saw the chapel that day last spring, I was reminded of it, and something made even more sense. But what made you run?" he asks her. "And into poison oak."

"I had just watched my father and my mother's lover fighting on the front lawn, and I had seen the neighbors watching, which was probably the source of my horror . . . now that I think about it. And I thought my father would punish me for watching. I'll let you tell me all the rest."

"No," he says. "I think I'm learning that I'm not going to tell you much—and maybe there's no need to anyway. I take it your parents are divorced?"

"Oh no, that would have been too sensible."

She moves beneath him and he raises his hips, but she pulls him back. He is struck by how quiet it is, how still, far quieter than his bit of residential real estate. "Do you ever leave the wall open?" he asks, looking into the gray foliage of the candle-light flickering on the wall.

"That would be too spooky."

"A little too much vastness?" he asks.

"Maybe," she says, and then he feels his own body surging and then all the space around him gathering itself into his body and then gathering even more tightly into her body beneath him.

She has been gone for hours already, but still he hears the sound of her, a resident volubility—it is not a house now from which her presence is ever leached. In the bathroom mirror, reflected, towels, their towels, what a color! He hates it; he loves it. It could not matter less; what matters is that it is their color, their towels hanging crookedly, one damp hours before the other, now both damp, together damp, their towels somehow the color of that first walk at Refugio, the color in the offing.

In the breakfast room, the table is mounded up in the middle with gourds, pumpkins, golden leaves, a few buckeyes, more than a few pods he cannot identify, though what he can identify, what does sound loudly here, is the eye that chose them, enshrined them here—Alice so strongly sonic, theatrical, scenic, this house now and its surfaces, its recesses full of Alice. He supposes this is true of most houses, what men despise in those days after separation, either the fact that she can still be heard or that what was once the tremendous sonic presence is now deafeningly silent. Why he would think about absence now in the midst of such presence, he does not know—and yet he knows. *And then there was no Sadie, no daughter, no sister. And then there was no father, no husband.* And then even Janey was somewhat attenuated, not there so much as companion, as surrogate daughter, and each time Luke's importance strengthened, engraved itself further—he knows about absence, what to do in its austerity, how to metamorphose into whatever space needs filling. It is presence he is learning to live beside.

He looks for a note, wants there always to be one, but she is erratic in this activity, and though he's not given it intense scrutiny, he can't find a pattern, any sense of displeasure when there's not a note, any sense of particular adoration when there is. Today there is no note, and when he determines this definitively—quick glances across the butcher block, the counters, the clip on the refrigerator—he settles the kettle on the stove, takes in the momentary, alarming nose of gas as he switches on the burner and likes—just likes—the blue flames gusting up against the black enamel bottom of the kettle.

It is Sunday again, their day, Luke thinks, though there are plenty of Sundays, like today, in which he works at home in his den, the house beyond him quiet, and yet this quiet very unlike the utter empty stillness he was used to. Alice is now here in this house, just not exactly here right now. Baptisms, christenings, breakfasts—they are often on Sundays—and she is gone to them early, preparing for them. On these Sundays, because she is usually home by late morning, they spend the rest of the day together, they cook, talk, do a bit of desultory work on the garden, mock horror at themselves: "We might as well be beavers or a swarm of locusts—look at this garden." But actually, the garden is flourishing. No resurrecting the plumerias, of course, but Luke bought three different colors of flowering maple, abutilon, the plant Alice had asked about that first evening at his mother's. He bought morning glories for himself, a few English roses, and a rare false cypress he had once seen in a pinetum in Delaware while at a conference. He'd done some research and found a nursery in South Carolina, but then he'd had to wrangle the shipping to Nevada, cajoling Louise into a trip to Las Vegas to pick it up. "Cannot ship to CA, ID, OR, or WA." Louise had been furious with him, endangering California agriculture, but then Luke reminded her she had not seen the Dale Chihuly ceiling of blown glass flowers at the Bellagio. "I'll pay for the entire trip. I'll even give you gambling change." And she had thrown a look at him and pronounced the word *change* with such derision that he thought for a moment she would not go. "Change," she said again, "change. Why would I go anywhere for *change*? I may be an old meter, but I have never run on change." Okay, okay, okay, and the tree—though he had ordered two, one for Louise also—had ended up costing him a couple thousand dollars, but his, or his and Alice's, stood handsomely in the yard—he is looking at it right now—its young, slender trunk, its soft drooping branchlets green and gold in the sunlight.

She will be home soon, but for the first time since they have lived together, he does not want her to be. Not just yet. He has been working most of the morning on distinguishing for the L.A. County Unified School District behaviors traditionally thought of as "sissyish," and often observed in autistics. He is gathering test stories from his files, actual exchanges and episodes with autistic subjects, and then discussing the social interpretations one might make if it were the speech or behavior of typical children. He wants in particular teachers to understand how incapable autistic children are of perceiving social convention. He wants to finish this project, and he is almost there. He wants to make a little dinner. He wants to shower. He has a bracelet from his mother and he wants to give it to Alice tonight. Why it must be tonight, he doesn't know, as he has had it now for some time, a few months really. He teases himself that he is ready to stay her eyes with a real chunk of jewelry, though he would not be giving it to her if it mattered one whit, which of course makes him want to give it to her all the more. Louise found its original box, and he has opened its fine blue leather and shut it too many times over the last few days, contemplating he does not exactly know what, but something, their life together, this gold bracelet that has always been in his life, adorning his mother's wrist. He is glad it is not the charm bracelet, the one Louise has claimed for Janey, its boisterously rude charms. Not that he's a prude. He remembers thinking, as a teenager, his mother pretty damn cool wearing that bracelet, its tremendous tinkling racket, more than occasionally some other mother's eye catching the Priapus with his not so tiny phallus, the dominatrix whip, the merry widow made of gold filigree, but this is not the one he wants for Alice. He wants the carefully tooled gold flowers for Alice, the beautiful Greek bracelet his father gave his mother years ago when Sadie and he were children. This August, Louise had bowed her head, worked the clasp, and slipped it from her wrist and puddled it in his hands, warm from her body, and heavy. "Here. Seems you'll be needing this," she murmured wryly.

"No, Mother, I don't *need* this, thank you very much," he said archly.

"Certainly it couldn't hurt," she retorted, and he smiles now thinking of her, how she knew it would be that bracelet he wanted, her most beautiful, really, and how she had given it up as though it were some modest trinket, not even given it up really, as there was no sense of sacrifice on her part to make him feel guilty, nor, he realized, any absurd commentary. What a funny old broad. She'd certainly never whipped off any of those bracelets before, and as he held it in his hands, she had gone upstairs and then returned after a time with the blue leather box, the jeweler's address in Athens in precise gold lettering inside its silk-lined lid. "You don't have any old beads, do you?" he asked her. "That you don't want." Louise looked at him strangely for a moment and then he told her about Polly, and about what he had done several months back by making a little room for her, and though he stops short of explaining that he feels it has to do with Polly's sense of physical cohesion, he tells her it matters to a little girl he treats. When Luke leaves that evening, he has two items, one the fine leather box holding the bracelet, and the other a small round basket heaped with beaded necklaces.

The light in his den is high and bright and warm. He is surrounded by mounds of files, stacks of journal issues. Something in the light, the blondness of the files makes him think even more about Polly. "She isn't," he says out loud to himself. She isn't emerging from imitative fusion, and as heartened as he had wanted to be, as heartened as he had *been* by the episode of the costume, Polly pulling it on, showing Stewart Markens, it remained an isolated event of abstraction. It does not seem to Luke now that Polly is getting better. He fears that she continues to swallow many of the beads she leaves his office with. He had hoped a gift of beads—beads coming from a source they had never before come from—might help develop her capacity for representation beyond her own physical body, but he had observed no distinction at work in Polly of late. His mother's beads had become as much a part of Polly's physical integrity as anything else on Polly's table. There is something, however, that he feels he has figured out, fathomed, and that is Jordan Markens's pregnancy, Polly watching her mother grow before her very eyes, take on this extra and tremendous and cumbersome dimension—and then lose it. Polly watched her mother's reedy body distort, take on a shape utterly different and obviously uncomfortable, and then what emerged deranged even further all of their lives. Luke thinks he knows that the *idea* of physical fragmentation which so threatens Polly derived from watching a pregnancy that resulted in Polly's life being so drastically changed, her room lost, her projects destroyed, her mother's availability further diminished. What's different, what is off by a degree, is that Polly thinks *she* is pregnant, that her own body will at some point result in a partition that will forever and even more deeply discourage her existence. Of course, she is not exactly wrong, this projection of her mother's procreative ability onto herself—she does have those abilities, just not yet—and isn't that typical of the healthiest children, the assumption of responsibility, of a vast agency, and much beyond their means. Luke sees Polly deeply recessed under the eaves of her blond curls. Why is it you back there, Polly, and not a thousand other little girls? He wonders what inabilities of imagination most people have that Polly doesn't and vice versa, and then he hears Alice's car in the drive and the soft gnashing of her car door as it closes. He pulls open his desk drawer and looks at the long blue leather box lying across a miasma of pens and staples and paper clips. He's sitting here in all his funk, but maybe that's just the way to give it to her. He listens to her in the house, her step across the kitchen tile, and then he can't hear her, and for a moment there is some quiet terror in that. He pushes shut his desk drawer, starts to rise from his chair, but she is there, tapping on the door and then moving it open, her face coming around into the room, then her bare feet, shuffling out some steps, doing a cha-cha. He taps the drawer pull. "There's something in there for you." She sits in his lap and pulls her legs and arms up and curls tightly into a ball against his chest. "Just you," she says. "Just you."

ACKNOWLEDGMENTS

I drew on several books in the writing of Luke's professional mind. The articles in *Autism and Asperger Syndrome*, edited by Uta Frith, were fascinating to me and what I derived from them in creating Luke is at once particular and impressionistic. Years ago, I read Bruno Bettelheim's *The Empty Fortress* and later, *The Uses of Enchantment*; these writings sustained my interest in the minds of children. Frances Tustin's *Autistic States in Children* interested me greatly at one point and influenced me in creating a therapist. Through the years I have read much of the writing of Oliver Sacks and some of the work of Temple Grandin. Thank you. At some point I read work by Leo Kanner, the psychiatrist who first named the syndrome "autism." Recently I've read several articles of ethyl mercury as being a possible cause of the increased rates of autism in America. The most significant of these articles was written by Dan Olmstead and titled "Mercury Rising."

The information that Henry Lutins gives Luke on crustacean endocrinology was taken verbatim from the fifth edition of *Integrated Principles of Zoology*, Cleveland P. Hickman, Jr., Frances M. Hickman.

The books *Flowers For All Seasons, Fall, Winter, Spring, Summer* by Jane Packer inspired my sense of what floral creations could be if allowed both simplicity and range. Thank you.

Sharon Dynak and the Ucross Foundation gave me cloister when I most needed time to complete this novel. Thank you for something I have never been granted before: Uninterrupted time to write; food at my door; beauty as far as the eye could see.

Through the years, and tirelessly, Varley O'Connor has read my work and kept me cheered. Then, not too long ago, something she said led me to the excavation of this novel from my garage and into the hands of Erika Goldman. For both of them, my gratitude is boundless.

I am surrounded by fine colleagues and fine friends and my family; I will thank you in person, though any of the felicities in these pages are due to you.